Fitness and Health

Fifth Edition

Brian J. Sharkey, PhD
University of Montana

Human Kinetics

Library of Congress Cataloging-in-Publication Data

Sharkey, Brian J.
  Fitness and health / Brian J. Sharkey.--5th ed.
    p. cm.
  Includes bibliographical references and index.
  ISBN 0-7360-3971-6
  1. Physical fitness. 2. Health. I. Title.

RA781 .S527 2001
613.7--dc21

2001039004

ISBN: 0-7360-3971-6

This book is a revised edition of *Physiology of Fitness,* published in 1990 by Human Kinetics.

Acquisitions Editor: Michael S. Bahrke, PhD; **Managing Editor:** Amy Stahl; **Assistant Editor:** Derek Campbell; **Copyeditor:** Barbara Walsh; **Proofreader:** Julie A. Marx; **Indexer:** Betty Frizzéll; **Permission Manager:** Dalene Reeder; **Production Manager:** Heather Munson; **Graphic Designer:** Nancy Rasmus; **Graphic Artist:** Dawn Sills; **Photo Managers:** Clark Brooks, Les Woodrum; **Cover Designer:** Jack W. Davis; **Photographer (cover):** D. Graham/H. Armstrong Roberts; **Photographer (interior):** Photos on pp. 93, 238, and 298 by Les Woodrum; all other photos by Tom Roberts unless otherwise noted; **Art Managers:** Craig Newsom, Carl Johnson; **Illustrator:** Mic Greenburg

Human Kinetics books are available at special discounts for bulk purchase. Special editions or book excerpts can also be created to specification. For details contact the Special Sales Manager at Human Kinetics.

Printed in China

10 9 8 7 6 5 4 3 2 1

Human Kinetics
Web site: www.humankinetics.com

United States: Human Kinetics
P.O. Box 5076
Champaign, IL 61825-5076
800-747-4457
e-mail: humank@hkusa.com

Canada: Human Kinetics
475 Devonshire Road Unit 100
Windsor, ON N8Y 2L5
800-465-7301 (in Canada only)
e-mail: orders@hkcanada.com

Europe: Human Kinetics
Units C2/C3 Wira Business Park
West Park Ring Road
Leeds LS16 6EB, United Kingdom
+44 (0) 113 278 1708
e-mail: hk@hkeurope.com

Australia: Human Kinetics
57A Price Avenue
Lower Mitcham, South Australia 5062
08 8277 1555
e-mail: liahka@senet.com.au

New Zealand: Human Kinetics
P.O. Box 105-231, Auckland Central
09-523-3462
e-mail: hkp@ihug.co.nz

To Barbara, the perfect companion for the long run.

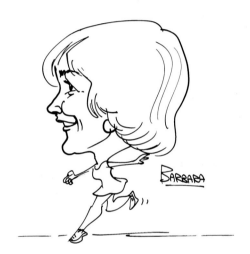

Contents

Preface

I was born in New York, was raised in New Jersey and Pennsylvania, and had just completed work on a doctorate in exercise physiology at the University of Maryland. Neither my wife nor I had ever ventured west of Harrisburg, Pennsylvania, until that day in 1964. On the first day of September we loaded two kids and some suitcases into our covered wagon, a Volkswagen sedan, and headed west to begin an academic appointment at the University of Montana. I had been hired over the phone, sight unseen, without a visit to the campus or the state. But I was happy to have a job, never imagining I would still be in the same place more than 35 years later. What took place, slowly but surely, was a subtle fusion of my academic interests with the magnificent geography and life of the mountain west. Before long I was hooked on the university, the mountains, and the active life. As our kids grew and we introduced them to the simple pleasures of active living, they responded with a deep sense of belonging in what has been called "the last best place."

After a few years I realized that Montana's long winter nights were ideally suited to writing. In 1968 I began a manuscript that emerged as my first book. Refined by several years of classroom use, *Physiological Fitness and Weight Control* was published in 1974. It provided sound advice for exercise and weight control, advice that, according to the Centers for Disease Control (USDHHS 1996), could save over 250,000 lives annually, then and now! This doesn't mean we haven't learned a great deal about physical activity, fitness, and health in the past two and a half decades. In fact, exciting research developments led me to author a retitled and expanded version of the original text in 1979, and then follow it with second and third editions in 1984 and 1990. The editions of that book, *Physiology of Fitness,* became a chronicle of new developments and my journey from fitness enthusiast to performance advocate and, finally, to a healthy respect for the benefits of the active life.

I tell you this to explain why I retitled the fourth (and now the fifth) edition to *Fitness and Health.* Epidemiological studies have shown that people can achieve many health benefits with regular moderate physical activity and can earn even greater rewards by improving their level of fitness. But the greatest gains, for personal and public health, come when individuals move from sedentary to active lifestyles. This edition affirms the importance of physical activity and fitness, highlighting one of the most exciting public health messages of our time.

Written for adults of all ages, this book is especially intended for the individual who wants to develop a deeper understanding of fitness and health, for the enthusiast who wants to know why and how the body responds, for the newcomer who needs motivation, and for the skeptic who needs proof. Years ago I set out to write the thinking person's fitness book; I hope you'll find that this edition meets that description.

Introduction to the Active Life

"Two roads
diverged in a
wood, and I—
I took the one
less traveled by,
And that has
made all the
difference."

Robert Frost

"When you
come to a fork
in the road . . .
take it."

Yogi Berra

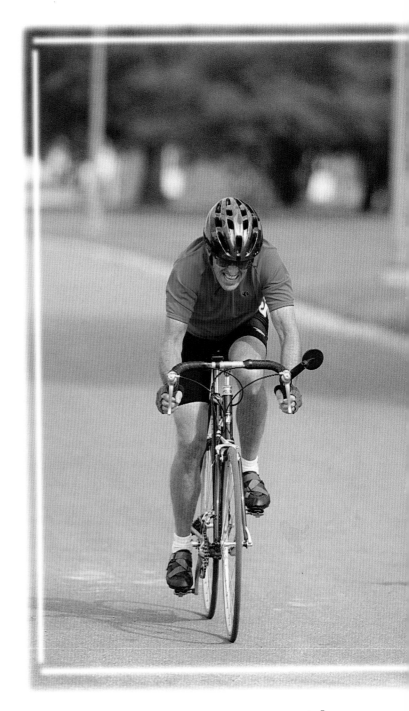

You've come to a fork in the road. One path shows evidence of heavy traffic, whereas the other—the one less traveled—is faintly etched upon the land. One travels downhill, the route of least resistance, while the other rises slowly to distant heights. Will you be seduced by the easy route or motivated by the high road and the view from above? Sadly, many choose the easy route, and as a consequence we Americans have lost our identity as a vigorous, vital people. Along the way we have become the fattest nation in the world, beset with chronic fatigue, depression, and degenerative diseases of the heart and lungs, of cancer and diabetes. My goal in writing this book is to convince you to take the road less traveled, knowing it will make all the difference in your life.

What is the road less traveled? Simply stated, it is the active life, a way of living based on regular physical activity and a cluster of related behaviors including healthy food choices, weight control, stress management, abstinence from tobacco and drugs, moderate use of alcohol, attention to safety (wearing seat belts and helmets), and disease prevention. It is the path of individual responsibility that leads not only to health, vigor, and vitality but also to self-respect and control of your destiny. This family of health-related behaviors has proven to be a profound paradox for our society, simple to comprehend but difficult to adopt.

The active life is the one people led before society achieved the benefits of industrial modernization: technological developments, the automobile, labor-saving devices, television, and computers. These marvels of ingenuity now make it possible to minimize daily energy expenditure by using buttons, keystrokes, and voice commands to meet survival, work, and entertainment needs. Parallel to the decline in the need for human energy expenditure has been an increase in the consumption of fatty, convenience, and fast foods. Food chemists added hydrogen to vegetable oils to prolong shelf (but not human) life and substituted low-cost palm and coconut oils for other ingredients to cater to our demand for tasty food in a hurry. Individually, the decline in activity or the rise in food consumption may not have been such a problem. Coming together as they have in recent years, the potential exists for alarming growth in the epidemic of diseases caused by the way we live. Fortunately, these behaviors can be changed.

This chapter will help you

- understand the dimensions of the active life,
- see how activity and other health behaviors interact,
- estimate activity levels in the population,
- define the amount of activity needed for health, and
- compare your current level of activity to recommended values.

Healthy Behaviors

The active life is at the core of a family of behaviors or habits that, viewed one at a time, seem too simplistic to be of much value. Yet collectively they are our greatest hope for personal health and vitality, and for the integrity of the nation's health care system. Many of the behaviors remind us of our mother's admonitions.

Healthy Habits

Some years ago researchers at the Human Population Laboratory of the California Department of Health published a list of habits associated with health and longevity (Breslow and Enstrom 1980). This list of habits included the following:

- Regular physical activity
- Adequate sleep
- A good breakfast
- Regular meals
- Weight control
- Abstinence from smoking and drugs
- Moderate use of (or abstinence from) alcohol

The study found that men could add 11 years to their lives and women 7 years just by following six of the seven habits.

Physical Activity

As many as 250,000 lives are lost annually because of the sedentary lifestyle.

The U.S. Centers for Disease Control and Prevention (CDC) and the American College of Sports Medicine (ACSM) reported that as many as 250,000 lives are lost annually because of the sedentary lifestyle (USDHHS 1996). If that sounds like an enormous number, you are right. Compare it to the number of lives lost annually in automobile accidents (under 50,000), from unprotected sexual intercourse (30,000), or from drug overdoses (20,000). Lack of physical activity is now considered as important a risk factor for heart disease as high blood cholesterol, high blood pressure, and cigarette smoking, not because activity is that potent, but because so many of us are inactive or sedentary. Inactivity contributes to a substantial number of the deaths from heart disease (34 percent) and costs $5.7 billion a year in medical costs (CDC 1993).

Healthy Food Choices

Poor food choices contribute directly to overweight, obesity, heart disease, diabetes, and cancer and indirectly to other problems such as depression. After years of health education, the average American still gets almost 40 percent of his or her daily calories from fat. In spite of all the books, newspaper and magazine articles, and television programs urging people to reduce fat intake to 30 or even 25 percent fat, the public seems surprised or confused about fat and cholesterol and about saturated and unsaturated fat. They seem unable to digest the important nutritional information printed on packages, information that clearly states the food's fat and cholesterol content. And far too few get the recommended daily servings of fruits and vegetables.

The World Is Fatter, Not Better Fed

Just because people are gaining weight does not mean the world is better fed or healthier, says the environmental group Worldwatch Institute. For the first time in history there are as many overweight as underfed people in the world, about 1.1 billion of each. In fact, being obese or underweight often results from the same problem: malnutrition. In the United States and other wealthier countries, the richer and the better-educated tend to eat right, whereas the poor often balloon from a diet of cheap and fatty fast foods. "Often, nations simply have traded hunger for obesity, and diseases of poverty for diseases of excess," said Worldwatch researchers. In the United States 55 percent of the population is overweight, with one in four adults considered obese (Associated Press, 3/5/2000).

Understanding the importance of nutrition and food choices becomes even more important as greater numbers of Americans enter the workforce; work longer hours; and rely more on convenience foods, take-home meals, and eating out. I'm lucky—I don't eat out that often, so when I do, it is a special event. At times I find it difficult to make healthy choices (such as fish rather than red meat); to avoid rich sauces, gravies, and desserts; and to eat in moderation. To avoid daily temptation I carry my lunch and eat at the desk after a vigorous workout. When I do eat out I ask for skim milk instead of whole, order dry toast, and request dressings served on the side. Along with healthy food choices, these changes in eating behavior are survival techniques for modern urban warriors. Poor diet, coupled with lack of exercise, causes at least 300,000 deaths a year, mostly from heart disease, and contributes to an increased risk of diabetes, cancer, and other ills.

Weight Control

Dieting for weight loss is the most unsuccessful health intervention in all of medicine.

Dieting for weight loss is the most unsuccessful health intervention in all of medicine. Only 10 percent of people who have lost 25 pounds or more will remain at their desired weight. Worse yet, many weight-loss programs contribute to obesity. The truth that has emerged from the last decade of research is that diet alone won't help you achieve permanent weight loss. What will? The active life, combined with healthy food choices, and behavior therapy if necessary, is the answer to lifelong weight control. Activity maintains or builds the lean tissue (muscle) that has the capability to burn calories. Diet, by itself, leads to the loss of muscle and a reduction in daily caloric expenditure, resulting in an increased storage of fat.

Stress Management

Stress is our emotional response to events in life. What one individual perceives as stress may be stimulating to another. Stress management implies the learning of effective coping strategies, or ways to deal with the many sources of stress in modern life. Stress has been linked to heart disease, cancer, ulcers, immunosuppression, and other ills. However, the link is uncertain due to the difficulty in measuring stress, and because some ills have been found to have other causes (e.g., ulcers are caused by bacteria). What is certain is that you can learn to cope

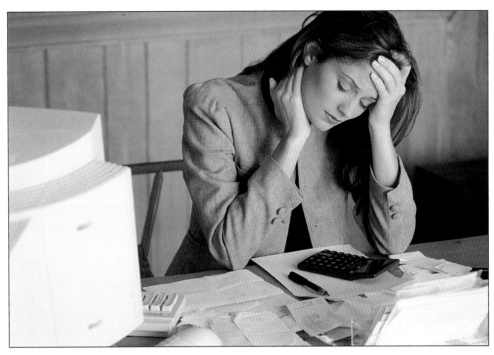

© Giovanni Lunardi/International Stock

Stress has been linked to heart disease, cancer, ulcers, and other ills.

with minor irritations and most major threats. The best results come when a person combines learned behavior changes with an arsenal of coping skills. Regular moderate activity is the ideal way to cope with stress because it is effective, long lasting, and much less expensive than drugs, and it provides other health benefits. As you'll see in chapter 2, activity can be psychologically therapeutic as well as preventive.

Other Healthy Behaviors

Another important aspect of the active life includes elimination of negative behaviors, such as addiction to tobacco and other drugs, and moderation in the use of alcohol. According to the Public Health Service's Office for Disease Prevention and Health Promotion, tobacco causes 400,000 deaths annually, including 30 percent of cancer deaths (85 percent of all lung cancer deaths) and 21 percent of cardiovascular deaths. Drug deaths total 20,000 per year, including overdose, suicide, homicide, AIDS (HIV infection), and more. Alcohol misuse causes 100,000 deaths a year, including almost half of all deaths from motor vehicle accidents (U.S. Department of Health and Human Services, Public Health Service 1991). And yet one or two drinks of alcohol each day, whether wine, beer, or the hard stuff, are associated with a reduced risk of heart disease. Who says disease prevention and health promotion have to be boring? One of the enjoyable little moments I experience daily is when I sit down to the evening news, a light beer, and some low-fat pretzels. The beer provides a tasty way to relax, reduce stress, and lower heart disease risk.

Safety habits such as the use of seat belts and child restraints in automobiles contribute to health and longevity. Bicycle and motorcycle helmets reduce the severity and cost of accidents. If cyclists want to feel the wind in their hair, they should be willing to bear the costs of long-term care associated with catastrophic

Combine personal responsibility with prevention and early detection tests, and you have a cost-effective strategy for survival.

accidents. Failure to use established safety devices should carry a cost for those who choose to ignore the need for personal responsibility.

The final category of health behaviors I want to mention is the habitual practice of preventive measures appropriate to your age, sex, medical condition, and family history. These measures include vaccinations and other preventive measures such as blood pressure and cholesterol checks; tests for glaucoma as well as prostate and breast cancer; and others. The fact is that you, not your doctor, are responsible for your health. Combine personal responsibility with prevention and early detection tests, and you have a cost-effective strategy for survival. The strategy is cost-effective because prevention is always cheaper than treatment, because you utilize lower-cost health providers, and because you need to see physicians less frequently. If your employer has a comprehensive employee health or wellness program, use it. If not, create your own as you assume personal responsibility for your health.

Key Point

By now you've noticed how many facets of the active life interact and overlap. Activity maintains muscle, which burns calories and fat; helps maintain a healthy weight; and reduces the risk of heart disease, diabetes, and cancer while it also serves as the centerpiece of the stress management program. Of course, it helps you look better as well. Healthy food choices (sometimes called good nutrition) help maintain or lose weight; lower cholesterol; reduce the risk of heart disease, cancer, and other ills; and make physical activity more enjoyable. The active life is not a hodgepodge of unrelated habits but rather a highly integrated family of behaviors that become more potent in combination than each is individually.

The Road Less Traveled?

According to the 1996 surgeon general's report, 25 percent of the population is sedentary and 60 percent is not regularly active. That leaves just 15 percent in the regularly active group (U.S. Department of Health and Human Services 1996). Thus, only 15 percent of the adult population is active enough to insure the physical and mental benefits of regular physical activity. The rest, a whopping 85 percent, deprive themselves of the joys and benefits of the active life and are likely to burden their families and the health care system. Sedentary habits vary by state, ranging from a low of 17 percent (Utah) to a high of 51 percent (Arizona). Recent overweight and obesity data suggest the rate of activity is declining. Indeed, the active life is the road less traveled. Isn't it time that you joined the ranks of the few, informed, resolute individuals who have the good sense and conviction needed to take the fork in the road, take personal responsibility, and embark on the active life?

Many view the active life and its associated behaviors as a medieval torture or religious rite, replete with fasting, denial, and mortification of the flesh. These folks are unwilling to give up the pleasures of rich (fatty) foods, unable to break addictions to tobacco, drugs, or alcohol. Since behaviors are often interrelated in a pattern of self-indulgence, these same individuals are likely to disdain the pleasures and rewards of the active life. Sadly, they do so at considerable cost to themselves and to society. For although few admit sorrow or repent their indulgences, they are destined to suffer a penance of fatigue and the purgatory of depression and disease. And the rest of us are expected to pay their bills and pick up the pieces of their lives.

Zealous fitness instructors have been heard to say, "No pain, no gain," "Go for the burn," or "It has to hurt to be good." Of course, none of these statements is true, unless you are involved in serious training for a highly competitive sport. And then the pain, the burn, and the hurt should be seen as identifiable end points during vigorous exercise. For most of us, pain, burn, and hurt need not be a part of our daily activity. The active life is not one of denial and deprivation, nor is it one of pain and suffering. It is a joyful experience, an affirmation of what we can be, physically, mentally, socially, and spiritually. It provides the energy to begin, the vigor to pursue, and the vitality to persist, to go the distance. It replaces overindulgence with moderation; substitutes positive for negative addictions; and yields health, energy, and the capacity to live.

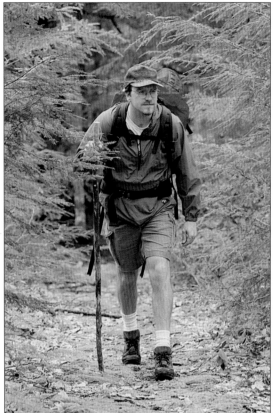

© The Terry Wild Studio Inc.

The active life is the road less traveled.

How Much Is Enough?

The public and some fitness instructors are confused. For years they thought that exercise had to be intense, as indicated by the mystical training heart rate, if it was to yield desired benefits. That recommendation still holds true if you are striving to improve your aerobic fitness. But what if your interest is in improving or maintaining health?

In the summer of 1993, a group of world-renowned experts came together with the ACSM and the CDC to develop new recommendations for physical activity and health. They reviewed the latest scientific evidence and reached consensus on the following recommendation:

- Every American adult should accumulate 30 minutes or more of moderate-intensity physical activity over the course of most days of the week.
- Because most adult Americans fail to meet this recommended level of moderate-intensity physical activity, almost all should strive to increase their participation in moderate or vigorous physical activity.

The recommendation suggests that a wide range of activities can contribute to the 30-minute total, including walking, gardening, and dancing. The 30 minutes (or more) of physical activity may also come from planned exercise or recreation, such as jogging, cycling, and swimming. The recommendation notes that a specific way to meet the standard is to walk two miles briskly. The ACSM/CDC recommendation tells those who currently do not engage in regular activity to begin with a few minutes of daily activity and build gradually to 30 minutes (Pate et al. 1995).

These recommendations are based on research that shows that adults who engage in regular moderate activity, enough to burn about 200 calories a day (e.g., brisk two-mile walk or jog), can expect many of the health benefits of exercise. From a public health perspective, we gain more if millions become active than we do if a few become superbly fit.

The Activity Index

Before we move on, you may want to gauge your current level of activity using this simple assessment tool. Developed in the 1970s, the index proved to be related to a laboratory test of aerobic fitness (the maximal oxygen intake). As you increase the intensity, duration, and frequency of exercise, your index score and fitness both go up. How much activity do you need? That is a decision you'll make as you become better acquainted with the pleasures and benefits of activity. A score of 40 or more on the activity index is an indication that you are active enough to earn many of the health benefits associated with physical activity. Increase the amount or intensity of exercise, and you will earn additional health benefits as you raise your aerobic fitness.

If your index score was below 40, you should begin today to increase your daily activity. Then, when we get into a discussion of the extra benefits associated with improved fitness, you will be ready to make a reasoned response to the question: "Am I satisfied with my current level of activity and fitness, or do I feel the need to undertake a training program?"

Summary

This chapter began with a description of the active life as the road less traveled, described how the health behaviors of the active life interact, and finished with a simple assessment of your level of activity. Along the way we documented the fact that less than 20 percent of the population is active enough to get the physical and mental benefits of regular activity, and we defined the amount of activity needed to achieve health benefits. This question remains: How did Americans reach such a dramatic level of inactivity?

We began as a vigorous nation of farmers, miners, loggers, laborers, and merchants; survived a revolution, a civil war, and the industrial revolution; migrated across the continent; and continued to thrive in spite of two world wars and a depression. Yet today, in spite of several decades of unparalleled economic development, we are gaining the reputation of being an overweight, lazy, complacent people, content to while away the hours with fast food, television, and video games. We have become the fattest nation in the world, with one-third of our adult citizens classified as obese. Our educational system is suffering from neglect, and we're the only developed country that has ignored the need for universal health

1

Health Benefits of Activity and Fitness

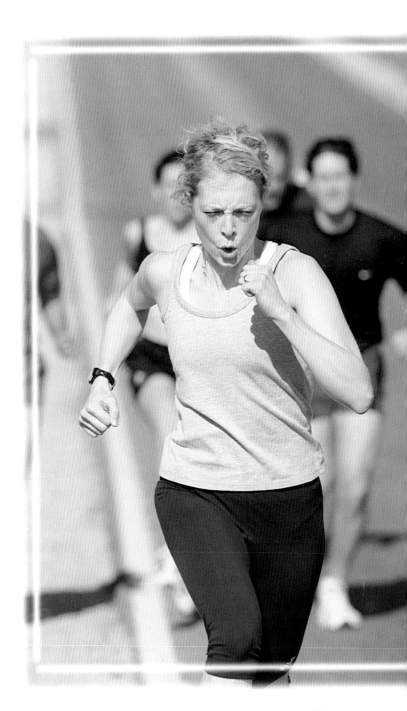

"Many of us spend half our time wishing for things we could have if we didn't spend half our time wishing."

Alexander Wollcott

The idea that physical activity is associated with good health is not new. The Chinese have long practiced a mild form of medical gymnastics to prevent diseases associated with lack of activity. In Rome more than 1,500 years ago, the physician Galen prescribed exercise for health maintenance. References to the health values of exercise can be found throughout recorded history, usually with little measurable effect on the populace. Why, then, do I invest time and energy in an effort to provide the latest evidence on the relationships between physical activity, physical fitness, and health? One reason is that I am a devout optimist, the product of more than 35 years of professional experience and many heart-warming success stories. Another reason is that never before have so many studies said so many good things about the health benefits of activity and fitness.

■ This chapter will help you

- understand the relationships among physical activity, fitness, and health;
- see how activity and fitness lower the risk of heart disease, hypertension, and stroke;
- appreciate how activity reduces the risk and severity of chronic diseases such as diabetes and some cancers;
- assess the role of activity in arthritis, osteoporosis, and low back problems; and
- understand how regular moderate physical activity contributes to the length and the quality of life.

Physical Activity, Fitness, and Health

Epidemiology, the study of epidemics, is a fitting way to study the modern epidemic—diseases of lifestyle—that is responsible for more than half of all deaths in the United States. The epidemiologist studies populations to determine relationships between behaviors, such as physical activity, and the incidence of certain diseases. Researchers look at morbidity (sickness) and mortality (death). Studies can be retrospective, looking back at past behaviors; cross-sectional, looking at chronological slices of the population; or prospective, following a group into the future. Retrospective studies are often troubled by lack of solid information on activity, fitness, and other health habits, while prospective studies face problems such as changing habits and participants who drop out. Most studies are plagued by issues of access to medical records (confidentiality), but the major problem is that of self-selection. Critics argue that subjects could be active because they are well, not necessarily well because they are active.

Because self-selection confounds the results of retrospective and cross-sectional studies, only carefully controlled prospective studies, involving random assignment of participants to levels of activity (or inactivity), allow cause-and-effect conclusions. Because these studies are difficult to conduct and most likely unethical (inactivity is dangerous to health), absolute proof of the value of activity and fitness may never be assembled. However, when the preponderance of studies support the health benefits of activity, and when the risks and costs are minimal, it seems reasonable to recommend a prudent—if not proven—course of action.

In that space does not permit a comprehensive review of the role of activity and fitness in health and disease, I will provide a summary of epidemiological findings and review several classic studies. To avoid endless details I will summarize the effects of activity and fitness with reference to the risk ratio (RR), the ratio of morbidity or mortality for the active members of the population to that for the inactive members. When possible I will indicate plausible mechanisms or reasons that activity may have beneficial effects, and I will conclude with a consideration of the risks and benefits of activity and recommendations for prudent behavior.

Risk Ratio

In a study of Harvard alumni, those with the least activity had 78.8 cardiovascular deaths per 10,000 versus 43 for the most active, yielding a risk ratio of 54 percent (43 divided by 78.8 equals .54). Stated another way, the risk was 46 percent lower (100 minus 54 equals 46 percent) for the active alumni (Paffenbarger, Hyde, and Wing 1986).

Activity and the Risk of Coronary Artery Disease

In spite of tremendous progress in the past 25 years, heart disease, or, more specifically, coronary artery disease (CAD), remains the nation's number-one killer for men and women. Heart, stroke, and blood vessel diseases kill almost one million people *in one year,* far more than all the lives lost in the four major wars of the last century (636,282). CAD is responsible for over half of those deaths, often in a sudden dramatic event called a heart attack. But this seemingly sudden event is actually the product of a process called atherosclerosis, a process that narrows the arteries and restricts the blood flow to the heart.

Atherosclerosis begins to develop during childhood, and the process is accelerated by a number of primary risk factors. In 1993, in recognition of the important role of activity, the American Heart Association (AHA) raised lack of physical activity to the level of the primary risk factors: cigarette smoking, elevated blood cholesterol, and high blood pressure (hypertension). Table 1.1 presents CAD risk factors and the possible influence of physical activity.

Table 1.1 CAD Risk Factors

Influenced by physical activity	May be influenced by physical activity	Not influenced by physical activity
Endomesomorphic body type	Insulin resistance	Family history of heart disease
Overweight	Electrocardiographic abnormalities	Gender (male has greater risk until 60s)
Elevated blood lipids	Elevated uric acid	Cigarette smoking
High blood pressure (hypertension)	Pulmonary function (lung) abnormalities	Diet (saturated fats, salt)
Physical inactivity	Personality or behavior pattern (hard driving, time conscious, aggressive, competitive)	
	Psychic reactivity (reaction to stress)	

Reprinted from Sharkey 1974.

Self-Evaluation: Do You Know Your Risk?

Do you have:

- ☐ High blood pressure (>140 mm Hg)?
- ☐ Elevated serum cholesterol (>240 mg)?
- ☐ Excess body weight?

Are you:

- ☐ A cigarette smoker?
- ☐ A bald male with a potbelly?
- ☐ Physically inactive?

To determine your health risk, complete the health risk analysis at the end of chapter 3.

Atherosclerosis may be initiated by inflammation of the lining of the coronary artery, a protective response to injury or even by an infection. Thereafter, high levels of circulating fats in the blood infiltrate the lining of the artery, aided perhaps by high blood pressure and chemicals, such as those in cigarette smoke. Low-density lipoprotein (LDL) cholesterol becomes oxidized, leading to further changes in the artery. A scablike plaque forms and grows until it blocks the flow of blood, or until the artery is clogged by a ruptured clot (figure 1.1). Some medical experts think viruses may accelerate atherosclerosis or stimulate immune system responses that contribute to plaque formation and clotting. Gradual narrowing reduces blood flow (ischemia) and often leads to exertional pain (angina) experienced in the chest, left arm, or left shoulder.

Some plaque is hard and some is soft; the soft plaque has the potential to burst and cause a clot that can interrupt blood flow and cause a heart attack (myocardial infarct). Lack of blood and oxygen can damage heart muscle if it isn't treated quickly. This soft, or "vulnerable," plaque may be the major cause of lethal heart attacks. The size, composition, and local inflammation processes may predispose a plaque to rupture. Biomechanical or hemodynamic forces, including increased blood pressure and heart rate; catecholamines; and even physical exertion sometimes precede and trigger rupture and the onset of an acute heart attack.

Autopsy studies show that atherosclerosis is under way in some young adults, and recent surveys have confirmed the presence of CAD risk factors in children of all ages. When doctors examined teenage hearts donated after accidental deaths, they found one in six already showed the blockage and plaque deposits characteristic of coronary artery disease (Tuzac 1999). Thus a program of risk factor identification and early intervention seems prudent, especially for those with a strong family history or multiple risk factors of heart disease. The active life can slow the process for many, and a demanding intervention program consisting of activity; a very low fat diet; and medication, if needed, may halt and even reverse the process (Ornish 1993).

Further proof of the extra benefits of fitness can be found in a study conducted in Finland. The authors concluded that higher levels of both leisure-time physical activity and fitness had a strong inverse relationship with the risk of heart attack. The study supports the conclusion that lower levels of physical activity and lower levels of fitness are independent risk factors for coronary artery disease in men (Lakka et al. 1994).

In Review

For now let me emphasize one of the most important public health messages of our time: Regular moderate physical activity conveys many if not most of the important health benefits associated with exercise. From a public health standpoint, an increase in physical activity will provide millions of Americans with some level of protection from heart disease, hypertension, adult-onset diabetes, certain cancers, osteoporosis, depression, premature aging, and more. Improved aerobic fitness provides added benefits. However, in both the Blair and Lakka studies, the level of fitness associated with extra benefits was not extremely high, and that level is therefore attainable by a large segment of the population. Indeed, epidemiologist Dr. Steven Blair has called low fitness caused by sedentary habits our *most important public health problem* (Blair 2000)!

Cardioprotective Mechanisms

Numerous studies have shown that physical activity and fitness are associated with a lower risk of CAD. Yet due to self-selection, most of the studies do not allow cause-and-effect statements and the level of assurance desired in scientific and medical research. To further investigate the influence of activity on cardiovascular health, researchers have explored a number of hypotheses concerning cardioprotective mechanisms (see table 1.3).

The major benefit of activity is its ability to metabolize fat and to lower circulating levels of fat in the blood.

Among the many possible ways in which activity may prevent or minimize the process of atherosclerosis, few are directly related to the heart itself. In my opinion, the major benefit of activity is its ability to metabolize fat and to lower circulating levels of fat in the blood (triglycerides and cholesterol). Let's explore some of these mechanisms to help explain why something as simple as regular moderate activity is so good for your health.

Activity's Effect on the Heart

Physical activity does have some direct effects on the heart, but not as many as you have been led to believe. Indeed, studies on the therapy called cardiac rehabilitation have been surprising in that they show little visible effect of exercise or training on the heart. Only when the training is prolonged and strenuous do we see measurable effects on the heart, and strenuous training may not reduce the risk of heart disease much more than moderate activity.

Efficiency of the Heart Regular activity reduces the workload of the heart. Changes in skeletal muscle, including improved oxygen-using (aerobic) enzymes and enhanced fat metabolism, allow the heart to meet exercise demands with a lower heart rate. The lower rate means a lower level of oxygen utilization in the heart muscle and a more efficient heart. Drugs are sometimes prescribed to lower

Table 1.3 Cardioprotective Mechanisms

Physical activity may

Increase	Decrease
Oxidation of fat	Serum cholesterol and triglycerides
Number of coronary blood vessels	Glucose intolerance
Vessel size	Obesity, adiposity
Efficiency of heart	Platelet stickiness
Efficiency of peripheral blood distribution and return	Arterial blood pressure
Electron transport capacity	Heart rate
Fibrinolytic (clot-dissolving) capability	Vulnerability to dysrhythmias
Arterial oxygen content	Overreaction to hormones
Red blood cells and blood volume	Psychic stress
Thyroid function	
Growth hormone production	
Tolerance to stress	
Prudent living habits	
Joy of living	

Reprinted from Sharkey 1974.

the workload of the heart, but activity and fitness are a more natural approach to the problem, without undesirable side effects.

Metabolic alterations associated with training may protect the heart during periods of inadequate blood flow (Libonati 1999). Some portion of the improvement in efficiency of the heart is due to improved contractility of the cardiac muscle, to diminished myocardial response to the oxygen-wasting hormone epinephrine (adrenaline), and to an increase in blood volume with training. If the heart pumps more blood each time it beats it doesn't have to beat as often. Regularly active and fit individuals have lower resting and exercise heart rates and a higher stroke volume (amount of blood pumped each beat).

Heart Size Because skeletal muscle gets larger with training, some have wondered if the same holds true for the heart. Studies of endurance training suggest that the trained heart is larger, but the increase is largely in the volume of the left ventricle, allowing a greater stroke volume. Subtle changes have been noted in the concentration of aerobic enzymes in heart muscle, which is not surprising in that the heart is already the ultimate endurance muscle. Those who do serious long-term resistance training experience some increase in the thickness of the heart muscle as it works to pump blood against the vascular resistance provided by contracting muscles. Exercise-induced cardiac hypertrophy, or the athlete's heart, is a healthy response to systematic training.

Blood Supply Studies show that activity improves the circulation within the heart. Animal and human studies suggest that in some but not all subjects, moderate activity enhances the development of coronary collaterals, alternative circulatory routes that help distribute blood and minimize the effects of narrowed coronary arteries. A fascinating effect of regular activity, first suggested after the autopsy on marathon runner Clarance DeMar, is an increase in the diameter of the coronary arteries, perhaps minimizing the effect of plaque formation. Kramsch and associates (1981) studied the effect of moderate exercise and an atherosclerotic diet on the development of CAD in monkeys. Electrocardiogram (ECG) changes and sudden death occurred only in the sedentary animals, whereas the exercise group had larger hearts and larger-diameter coronary arteries.

Activity's Effect on the Vascular System

The following mechanisms suggest ways that activity may lower the risk of CAD via changes in or within the blood vessels. They include beneficial changes in blood clotting, blood pressure, and blood distribution.

Blood Clotting   Blood is designed to form a clot and stem the flow of blood when we are injured. But a clot (called a thrombus) that forms within an uninjured vessel is dangerous, and a clot in a narrowed coronary artery could be disastrous. Clots form when the soluble protein fibrinogen is converted to insoluble threads of fibrin. Normally we are able to dissolve an unwanted thrombus by dissolving the fibrin (fibrinolysis). Exercise enhances this process, but the effect lasts only a day or two. The stress of exhaustive or highly competitive exercise seems to inhibit this system, allowing a more rapid clotting time. Regular, moderate, or even vigorous activity is the way to enhance the body's ability to dissolve unwanted clots (Molz et al. 1993). In fact, a review of the literature concluded that regular exercise is the most practicable approach known to date to lower plasma fibrinogen levels (Ernst 1993).

Aspirin

Studies have shown that one aspirin a day (or one every other day) reduces the risk of unwanted clots associated with heart disease and stroke. The aspirin reduces the stickiness of platelets, small particles in the blood that get caught in the fibrin threads of a developing clot. One aspirin a day, taken with a meal, is tolerated by most folks. It is an inexpensive way to reduce the risk of CAD and stroke, and it may also help reduce the risk of colon cancer.

Blood Pressure   High blood pressure, or hypertension, increases the workload of the heart by forcing it to contract against the greater resistance. Anything that lowers blood pressure also reduces the workload of the heart. Regular moderate physical activity has been shown to reduce blood pressure in middle-aged or older individuals. And walking, but not weightlifting, has been shown to reduce systolic blood pressure in elderly individuals (Rejeski et al. 1995). Recent studies suggest that regular activity may help maintain the elasticity of blood vessels in aging subjects. Of course, changes in blood pressure could also be the consequence of weight loss or reduced stress, both known outcomes of regular activity.

Blood Distribution   Regular physical activity teaches the body to better distribute the blood to muscles during exercise, further reducing the workload of the heart. Constricting vessels leading to digestive and other organs and dilating vessels that serve working muscles allow the blood to flow where it is needed. Of

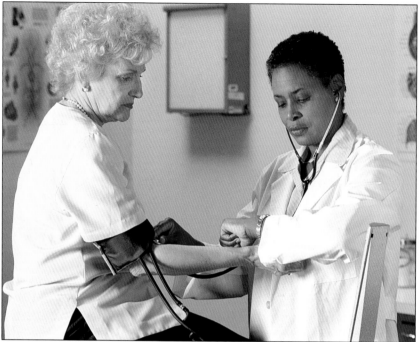

Regular moderate physical activity has been shown to reduce blood pressure.

course, the 10 to 15 percent increase in blood volume that comes with endurance training further enhances the performance of both the heart and skeletal muscles. These changes serve to lower the heart rate and blood pressure during physical activity. Because the oxygen needs of heart muscle are directly related to the product of heart rate and blood pressure, these improvements serve to reduce the likelihood that you'll exceed the ability to supply oxygen to cardiac muscle. As with most other effects of activity and training, the benefits depend on regular, not occasional, activity.

Metabolic Changes Due to Activity

This package of metabolic mechanisms may be the most important in the fight against CAD as well as several other disorders.

Fat Metabolism Eat too much and you gain weight in the form of stored fat. Excess fat is a health risk for heart disease, hypertension, diabetes, and some forms of cancer. You can diet (starve) to get rid of fat, but there is a hitch: The starving breaks down muscle tissue for energy, so you lose the only tissue that is capable of burning large amounts of fat. Muscular activity is the proven way to mobilize fat from adipose tissue storage, and then to burn it for energy in skeletal muscles. Exercise burns fat and avoids loss of muscle protein; in fact, regular activity can build additional muscle, thereby enhancing your ability to burn fat.

Regular activity burns calories, helping you to maintain a desirable body weight and percent body fat and a leaner, healthier figure. Fitness training leads to an enhanced ability to mobilize and metabolize fat. The physically fit individual is the owner of an efficient fat-burning furnace. This enhanced ability to utilize fat as an

The physically fit individual is the owner of an efficient fat-burning furnace.

energy source leads to even greater benefits that are closely tied to a reduced risk of atherosclerosis and CAD. Physical activity has even been found to decrease the risk of developing gallstones, independent of other risk factors such as obesity and recent rapid dietary weight loss (Leitzmann et al. 1999).

Blood Lipids   Lipid is another word for fat; the blood lipids include cholesterol and triglycerides, and each is related to the risk of heart disease. The level of cholesterol in the blood is an important predictor of the risk of heart disease. Total cholesterol includes low-density lipoprotein (LDL) cholesterol and high-density lipoprotein (HDL) cholesterol. Regular activity can lead to a modest decline in total cholesterol, but that is only part of the story. LDL is the dangerous subfraction of cholesterol found in the plaques that clog coronary arteries. Activity, diet, and weight loss all contribute to a drop in LDL. Regular activity, particularly vigorous activity, and weight loss both contribute to a rise in HDL cholesterol, the beneficial subfraction that collects cholesterol from the arteries and transports it to the liver for removal from the body. So exercise reduces total cholesterol (especially the LDL portion), raises HDL, and greatly improves your cholesterol/HDL ratio, one of the best predictors of heart disease risk.

Cholesterol/HDL Ratio

Before training and weight loss, Bill had a cholesterol level of 240 and an HDL of 40, for a ratio of 240 divided by 40, or 6, and a moderately high risk of CAD. Training and weight loss reduced the cholesterol to 200 and raised the HDL to 50, yielding a much-improved ratio of 4. He could continue to improve his lipid profile and further reduce his risk of CAD by continuing the fitness training, maintaining his body weight, and reducing his consumption of total and saturated fat. I'll say more about cholesterol in later chapters.

Triglycerides, consisting of three fatty acids and a molecule of glycerol, constitute a transport and storage form of fat. High levels are associated with heart disease, obesity, and hypertension. Regular activity is a proven way to lower circulating levels of triglycerides. Levels are reduced several hours after exercise, and the effect persists for one or two days. Several days of exercise lead to a progressive reduction of triglyceride levels. The final plateau depends on the diet, body weight, the intensity and duration of exercise, and one's genetic tendency. It is clear that regular moderate activity leads to a significant reduction in triglycerides.

Other Metabolic Mechanisms   A number of additional metabolic mechanisms support the value of activity as a cardioprotective therapy. Regular activity and training have been shown to increase insulin sensitivity and glucose tolerance. This effect of exercise is particularly important for individuals who are obese and those with adult-onset diabetes (also called type II diabetes or non-insulin-dependent diabetes mellitus—NIDDM). High levels of circulating fat inhibit insulin's ability to help transport glucose into muscles. Exercise enhances the transport, even in the absence of insulin. Thus, regular activity helps by reducing body weight and fat levels and by increasing insulin sensitivity and glucose transport. All these improvements reduce the risk of heart disease and NIDDM.

Metabolic Syndrome

Defined as a clustering of metabolic abnormalities related to insulin resistance and hyperinsulinemia, metabolic syndrome, which has also been called "the deadly quartet," includes the following:

- Blood pressure >140 mm Hg
- Serum triglycerides >150 mg
- Fasting blood glucose >110 mg/dl
- Central adiposity (waist circumference >39.3 in [100 cm])

This cluster of metabolic markers is associated with obesity, diabetes, and heart disease. Low levels of cardiorespiratory fitness are associated with increased clustering of the metabolic abnormalities of the syndrome in adult men and women (Whaley et al. 1999).

Electrolytes Electrolytes, including potassium, sodium, and calcium, are essential to the function of muscles, including the heart. During exertion the untrained heart may experience a diminished oxygen supply, which can trigger an imbalance of electrolytes, electrical instability, and disturbances in heart rhythms. Death can result from lethal rhythm disorders, such as tachycardia (rapid beating) or fibrillation (irregular, uncontrolled, unsynchronized beating). Fitness training minimizes this likelihood by reducing the heart's workload, improving oxygen supply and efficiency, and correcting electrolyte imbalances.

Psychological Stress

Most folks and some researchers are convinced that stress, or our reaction to it, is a major factor in the development of atherosclerosis and CAD. Years ago Friedman and Rosenman (1973) identified the Type A personality as a risk factor characterized by competitiveness, ambition, and a profound sense of time urgency. They claimed that among the subjects in their studies, Type As had a greater incidence of CAD. Analysis of the Framingham study (Wilson, Castelli, and Kannel 1987), a longitudinal study of an entire community, failed to find a link between stress and heart disease. This could be because stress is hard to measure with a paper-and-pencil test. Recent work in this area suggests that anger and repressed hostility are related to heart disease, and that Type A behavior by itself does not pose a problem. Others are searching for "hot reactors," those angry, hostile individuals who have exaggerated increases in blood pressure and stress hormones when faced with daily events (e.g., road rage).

Though meditation and other forms of stress management are useful, regular moderate activity is the best form of stress management.

I do know that regular activity is a coping mechanism that serves to improve tolerance to psychological stress. Though meditation and other forms of stress management are useful, regular moderate activity is the best form of stress management. Why? Because it provides the benefits of meditation and relaxation while it delivers added health benefits, including weight loss; reduced risk of CAD, hypertension, cancer, diabetes, and other ills; control of anxiety and depression; and improved appearance, vitality, even longevity. I'll say more about stress in chapter 2.

Physical Activity Reduces the Risk of Chronic Diseases

I've taken a lot of time and space to establish the role of activity and fitness in reducing the risks of heart disease. Now I will briefly sketch how activity can protect you from an impressive list of chronic diseases and disorders.

Hypertension and Stroke

Individuals with high blood pressure (>160/95) are three times more likely to experience CAD and four times more likely to get congestive heart failure than others. Hypertension also increases the risk of stroke and kidney failure. The causes of hypertension are still under investigation. But we do know that inactivity increases the risk of developing hypertension by 35 percent, and that unfit subjects have 52 percent greater risk than the fit. Regular endurance exercise lowers systolic and diastolic pressures about 10 mm Hg. Active hypertensive patients have half the risk of death from all causes than inactive hypertensives (Paffenbarger 1994).

A stroke, a clot or hemorrhage of a blood vessel in the brain, can result in loss of speech or muscle control or even death. The risk factors are similar to those for CAD. In most studies the risk of stroke decreases as activity increases. However, with more vigorous activity, and possibly heavy lifting, the trend may reverse. Transient ischemic attacks (TIAs) are sudden, brief periods of weakness, vertigo, loss of vision, slurred speech, headache, or other symptoms that sometimes precede a stroke. Similar symptoms have been associated with heavy weightlifting exercises. Time and again we find compelling arguments for moderation.

Cancer and Immunity

In recent years, evidence that the active lifestyle is associated with a lower risk of certain types of cancers has been accumulating. Most often studied is the link between activity and a lower risk of colon cancer. Some researchers hypothesize that regular activity shortens intestinal transit time for potential carcinogens in the fecal material. If that is the mechanism, it is hard to understand why the incidence of rectal cancer isn't lower as well. A few studies suggest that activity may help reduce the risk of prostate cancer.

Women who were active in their youth have fewer cancers of the breast and the reproductive system (Frisch et al. 1985). These authors noted that body fat was lower in the previously active women. In fact, a more recent study of more than 25,000 women found that the risk was lowest (RR, or risk ratio, = .28) in lean women who exercised at least four hours per week (Thune et al. 1997). The role of dietary fat and obesity in the development of cancer continues to interest researchers.

Cancers may be initiated by a substance that causes genetic damage (e.g., by carcinogens in meat or cigarette smoke). Then promoters (such as estrogen in the case of breast cancer) stimulate cell proliferation. The healthy immune system may play a role in the control of initiators or in the suppression of transformed cells or their by-products. On the other hand, a compromised immune system may allow initiation and promotion to go unchecked. Regular moderate physical activity enhances the function of the immune system, whereas high levels of stress or exhaustive exercise seem to suppress the system.

Diabetes and Obesity

Researchers have begun to suspect a link between NIDDM, CAD, and hypertension, specifically that all three share insulin resistance and that obesity and lack of activity are part of the problem. Insulin-resistant cells can't take in glucose, so glucose levels rise and the body secretes more insulin, which tends to increase blood pressure (via increased blood volume and vasoconstriction). Obesity and high levels of blood lipids seem to foster a resistance to insulin, whereas exercise increases insulin sensitivity and the movement of glucose into working muscles. Regular activity has returned to a place of prominence in the treatment of NIDDM, and for some it removes the need for insulin substitutes. In general, regularly active adults have a 42 percent lower risk of NIDDM (RR = .58).

Arthritis, Osteoporosis, and Back Problems

This group of musculoskeletal problems accounts for significant pain and suffering, as well as billions of dollars for often unnecessary treatments. All of these problems can be treated or prevented with activity. Arthritis isn't caused by exercise unless there is a previous injury. And regular moderate activity is an essential part of the treatment.

Osteoporosis is the progressive loss of bone mineral that occurs faster in women, especially after menopause. It is accelerated by cigarette smoking, low body weight—especially from dieting—and lack of activity. With age the condition can lead to brittle bones, hip fractures, and the characteristic dowager's hump caused by the collapse of vertebrae in the neck. The bone mineral loss can be slowed with adequate calcium intake, regular weight-bearing exercise, and, if necessary, hormonal therapy after menopause.

Back problems result from the acute or chronic assault to underused and undertrained bodies. The risk can be minimized or rehabilitated with regular attention to abdominal exercises and flexibility of the back and hamstring muscles. Among the many therapies used on back problems, including surgery, manipulation, injections, and drugs, none has been proven more effective than a rapid return to physical activity. I'll provide specific suggestions for back health in chapter 10.

Physical Activity Increases Longevity

By decreasing the risk of CAD, cancer, and other diseases of lifestyle, regular activity extends the period of adult vigor and compresses the period of sickness that precedes death. In a real sense, activity adds life to your years, and now there is evidence that it can also add years to your life. When Paffenbarger (1994) analyzed the effects of changing to more favorable health habits, moderate activity (1,500 calories per week) conferred an average of 1.57 years above less active living, and vigorous sports provided 1.54 years over no sports participation. Data on Harvard alumni indicated that vigorous activity (defined as more than 6.5 to 7.5 calories per minute, the equivalent of a brisk walk) was associated with reduced mortality. Mortality declined with increasing levels of vigorous activity up to about 3,500 calories per week, but not for nonvigorous activity (Lee, Hsieh, and Paffenbarger 1995).

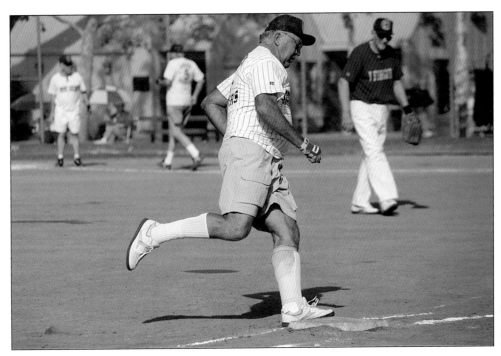

© Mary Messenger

Activity adds life to your years.

A report from the Institute for Aerobics Research (Blair et al. 1995) confirmed the fact that fit folks live longer. Based on 9,777 men aged 20 to 82, the data showed that men who were unfit when they entered the study were 44 percent less likely to die over the 18-year period of the study if they improved their fitness. Those who were fit at the start of the study and remained fit were 67 percent less likely to die than those who remained unfit. The benefits were found across all age groups, and the most fit individuals had the lowest risk of premature death. I'll say more about aging and how to live better and longer in chapter 18.

Waging War on Chronic Diseases

In an attempt to develop a new approach to research on physical activity, and to counter the epidemic of chronic diseases that emerged in the latter part of the 20th century, researchers have recommended a novel approach to the problem. They argue that the human genome evolved within an environment of high physical activity. Accordingly, they propose that researchers do not study the "effect of physical activity" but instead study the effect of *reintroducing* exercise into an unhealthy, sedentary population that is genetically programmed to expect activity (Booth et al. 2000). The authors argue that a major redirection of research funding will be needed to avoid bankruptcy of the U.S. health care system, and that a significant amount must be spent to study primary prevention of chronic diseases and the role of physical activity and fitness.

"That the richest country in the world is willing to spend billions of dollars in medical costs for some diseases that might be ameliorated by truly vigorous and sustained efforts aimed at making moderate regular physical activity part of every American's life-style is one of these inconsistencies that has been our collective heritage."

Roberta Park

Summary

For 50 years epidemiologists have studied the relationships of occupational and leisure-time activity with health, and an impressive list of benefits has emerged. The studies clearly show how activity enhances health while it reduces the risk of CAD, hypertension, and stroke as well as some cancers, diabetes, osteoporosis, obesity, and other chronic disorders. I've presented evidence of additional health benefits associated with vigorous activity and fitness and shown how regular moderate physical activity extends the length and the quality of life. Now we will turn our attention to the topic of psychological health, to see how the active life contributes to mental health and the joy of living.

2

Activity and Mental Health

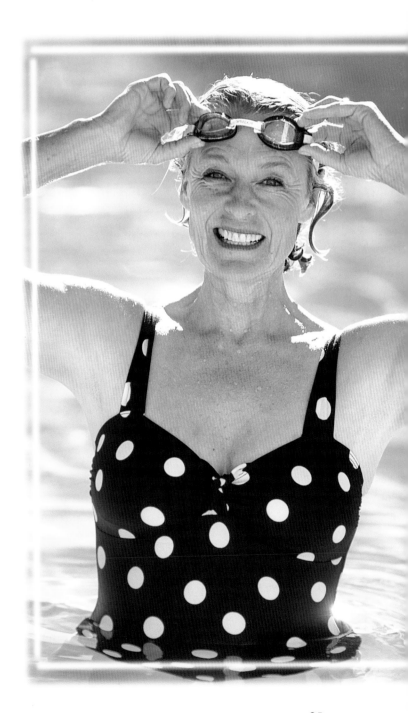

"A sound mind in a sound body is a short but full description of a happy state in this world."

John Locke

Everyone has heard of psychosomatic illness, a physical ailment caused or exacerbated by the state of mind. But few have heard the term somatopsychic, which suggests the effect of the body (soma) on the mind. This chapter describes how use of the body, specifically with regular moderate physical activity, has a beneficial effect on the mind and mental health. Although the research in this area is still in its infancy and many questions remain, it is important to review the case for what may be the most important role for activity and fitness.

As with activity and physical health, we must wonder about self selection: Does activity promote mental health, or does mental health promote activity? Do happy, less anxious, and nondepressed individuals have the interest, vigor, and energy to be active? Evidence from epidemiological studies indicates that the level of physical activity is positively associated with good mental health, when mental health is defined as positive mood, general well-being, and relatively infrequent symptoms of anxiety and depression (Stephens 1988). And as you will see, in intervention studies, activity has been associated with reduced levels of anxiety and depression. If it is true, as some have estimated, that at any given time as many as 25 percent of the population suffer from mild to moderate anxiety, depression, and other emotional disorders, we should not ignore the potential of this safe, low-cost therapy.

This chapter will help you

- understand how activity reduces anxiety and depression,
- appreciate how activity helps us deal with stress, and
- recognize positive aspects of an addiction to activity.

Activity Reduces Anxiety and Depression

If activity were a drug, and it could be proven effective in the prevention and treatment of anxiety and depression, it would be hailed as a modern miracle, worth billions to the company with legal rights to the formula. Well, activity isn't a drug, but rather a learned behavior that requires the motivation to begin and the persistence to adhere to a program. This chapter deals with mental health problems, while chapter 19 provides the psychological support you'll need to begin and continue the active life.

Anxiety

Anxiety has been defined as a diffuse apprehension of some vague threat, characterized by feelings of uncertainty and helplessness. It is more than ordinary worry in that it can be perceived as a threat to one's self-esteem. *State anxiety* is a transitory emotional response to a very specific situation. It is characterized by feelings of tension, apprehension, and nervousness. *Trait anxiety* is considered a relatively stable level of anxiety proneness, a predisposition to respond to threats with elevated anxiety. Studies have investigated the effects of acute and chronic activity on state and trait anxiety.

Activity such as walking has been shown to reduce state anxiety, as have meditation, biofeedback, and some other forms of mental diversion. So if you are tense and apprehensive about an upcoming responsibility, meeting, or presenta-

known as the runner's high. Although blood endorphin levels are elevated during and after an endurance effort, studies have shown that the levels do not correspond with mood states (Markoff, Ryan, and Young 1982). It isn't surprising, though, that blood levels and moods might not correlate, because a blood-brain barrier prevents easy transport between the systemic circulation and the brain. Hence, blood levels of endorphins do not tell us what is happening to endorphin levels in the brain, where moods are formed. The increased levels in the blood are probably a reflection of endorphins' role as a narcotic. Running feels easier after about 20 minutes, which is when increased levels of beta endorphin have been detected. So if you have tried running and found it uncomfortable, try to continue beyond 20 minutes; you may find it becomes easier with the help of your natural painkillers.

Acidosis?

An interesting study correlated a number of measures to beta endorphin release during exertion. Surprisingly, the level of lactic acid in the blood was one of the measures most associated with endorphins, suggesting that strenuous effort that produces lactic acid is more likely to lead to their release. When the acid was buffered during exertion, endorphin release was suppressed (Taylor et al. 1994).

It is clear that activity and fitness have the potential to improve mild to moderate cases of anxiety and depression. But why wait until you are anxious or depressed to begin? Start now, and you may be able to prevent or minimize these assaults on your mental health.

Activity and Stress

Many believe that stress has become one of the modern age's major health problems. Physiological responses necessary for the survival of primitive peoples may be unhealthy in highly complex societies. Stress, tension, and reactive behavior patterns have been associated with heart disease, hypertension, suppression of the immune system, and a variety of other ills. The emotional response to life events is mediated by structures in the brain, including the hypothalamus. When something excites or threatens us, the hypothalamus tells the anterior pituitary gland to secrete adrenocorticotropic hormone (ACTH), a chemical messenger that travels to the adrenal cortex and orders the release of hormones such as cortisol. These hormones are necessary for the body's response to stressful situations. Without them the body cannot deal with stress; it collapses and dies. Stress has been defined as anything that increases the release of ACTH or cortisol.

Type A

The Type A behavior pattern is characterized by extreme competitiveness, ambition, and a profound sense of time urgency. The Type B personality, the opposite of the Type A, is relaxed, calm, even phlegmatic. In studies by cardiologists Friedman and Rosenman (1973), Type A subjects had higher cholesterol levels, faster blood clotting times, higher adrenaline levels, more sudden deaths, and a sevenfold greater risk of heart disease. Subsequent studies, including the massive Framingham study, failed to find a link between the Type A behavior pattern, stress, and heart disease. They did find a link between anger, repressed hostility, and heart disease risk (Wilson, Castelli, and Kannel 1987).

Though most of us intuitively accept stress as a risk factor for heart disease, the Type A personality, in the absence of anger and hostility, does not seem to be a problem. Studies of the corporate structure suggest that it is the employees, not the hard-driving executives, who face the most stress. Executives live fast-paced lives but retain a sense of control. Employees often feel they have no control over their lives, and that is stressful.

Stressful situations also elicit a response in the sympathetic nervous system that leads to secretion of hormones from the adrenal medulla, including epinephrine (adrenaline) and norepinephrine. These hormones mobilize energy and support the cardiovascular response to the stressor. This aspect of the stress response is called the fight-or-flight mechanism. The hormones prepare the body to fight or run, but they have other effects that can be bad for the health. Epinephrine makes the blood clot faster, an advantage in a fight but a disadvantage in the workplace, where it can precipitate a heart attack or a stroke.

The stress response is necessary to prepare an athlete for a maximal effort in a race or physical challenge, but it can be unhealthy if it occurs too often in the wrong setting. If you become stressed on the job, when a natural physical catharsis is impossible or improper, the circulating hormones can be a problem. Recent research has suggested that some of us are hot reactors, exhibiting exaggerated blood pressure responses to everyday stressors. Hot reactors become enraged when a driver cuts them off in traffic (road rage), or as a result of other psychosocial stressors. This hostility elicits a flood of hormones designed for combat. Blood pressure and heart rate increase, arteries constrict, and clotting time shortens, contributing to an increased risk of a coronary. Hot reactors stew in their own juices, setting the stage for immediate or future health problems. Prolonged exposure to stress hormones eventually suppresses the immune system, and reduced resistance to infection is a sign of stress.

Some early rat studies suggested that exercise itself was a stressor (Selye 1956). Those results make sense when you realize that the animals were forced to run on a treadmill and were shocked when they tried to rest, or forced to swim to exhaustion in a deep tank with a weight tied around the tail. Electroshock and fear of drowning are stressful for most of us. For humans, exercise is stressful when it is highly competitive, exhausting, or threatening. Rock climbing, for example, is stressful for the neophyte and exhilarating for the veteran. Stress is in the eye of the beholder.

Regular moderate activity minimizes the effects of stress. It is relaxing and tranquilizing and has been shown to counter the tendency to form blood clots. Regular activity enhances the function of the immune system, whereas the exhaustion of a marathon is immunosuppressive. Occasional exposure to stressful activity is fine if you have trained for the event. Regular moderate activity and fitness contribute to your health, in part by reducing the diastolic blood pressure response to stress (Hendrix and Hughes 1997).

Stress is in the eye of the beholder.

Stress Test

Certain life events, both positive and negative, have been identified as stressful. A score of over 300 points in the past year has been associated with a serious illness within two years. Here are some of the events and their relative stressfulness.

Death of spouse	100 points
Divorce	73
Separation	65
Jail term	63
Death of family member	63
Personal injury or illness	53
Marriage	50
Fired from job	47
Retirement	45
Marital reconciliation	45
Pregnancy	40
Death of friend	37
Mortgage	31
Personal achievement	28
Spouse starts/stops work	26
Trouble with boss	23
Change of residence	20
Vacation	13

If life is getting too stressful, slow the pace of change (Roth and Holmes 1985).

If life is getting too stressful, slow the pace of change.

Psychoneuroimmunology

A relatively new area, psychoneuroimmunology (PNI), studies links between the brain, the nervous system, and the immune system. PNI focuses on how thoughts, emotions, and personality traits interact with the immune system and become manifest in sickness or health. Thoughts or emotions can enhance or suppress the immune system via neurotransmitters secreted by the sympathetic nervous system, or via hormones released upon command of the brain (e.g., ACTH). The immune system is immensely complicated, consisting of lymphocytes, T cells, natural killer cells, antibodies, immunoglobulins, and more. It serves to protect the body from foreign assaults. When exposed to prolonged stress, however, the system tends to break down, allowing invading microorganisms to proliferate. PNI suggests that by altering your perception of the supposed threat, by reprogramming your thinking and your outlook on life, you can reduce exposure to stress and spare the immune system.

Another way to bolster the immune system is with regular activity. Recent studies confirm the beneficial effect of activity and training on components of the immune system. The studies agree that regular moderate activity and training contribute to a healthy immune system (Mackinnon 1992; Nieman and Pedersen 1999). Excessive intensity, duration, or frequency of training risks overtraining, a condition characterized by fatigue, poor performance, and suppression of the immune system. Activity, relaxation, imagery, and other coping strategies help you deal in a rational way with difficult problems, freeing the immune system to function on your behalf.

Activity and Addiction

Substance abuse with nicotine, alcohol, or prescription or recreational drugs presents a health and social dilemma of such dimensions it threatens to tear society apart. Each of these substances presents a staggering cost in health care, rehabilitation, and social services, not to mention the loss of human potential. I don't pretend to have answers to this national problem, but I do have some suggestions for prevention and individual responsibility.

In his book *Positive Addiction,* Dr. William Glasser contrasts positive and negative addictions (1976). Negative addictions such as drugs or alcohol relieve the pain of failure and provide temporary pleasure but at a terrible cost in terms of family, social, and professional life. Positive addictions lead to psychological strength, imagination, and creativity. Dr. Glasser suggests that as an individual participates in meditation, yoga, or running, he or she eventually achieves the state of positive addiction. When this state is reached the mind is free to become more imaginative or creative. The mind conceives more options in solving difficult or frustrating problems; it has more strength. Proof of addiction comes when you are forced to neglect your habit, and guilt and anxiety accompany the early stages of withdrawal.

Positive Addiction

Positive addiction can be achieved from almost any activity you choose, as long as it meets the following criteria:

- It is not competitive.
- You do it for approximately one hour daily.
- It is easy to do and doesn't take much mental effort.
- You can do it alone or occasionally with others, but you don't rely on others to do it.
- You believe it has some physical, mental, or spiritual value.
- You believe that if you persist you will improve.
- You can do it without criticizing yourself.

In the chapter entitled "Running—the Hardest But Surest Way," Dr. Glasser suggests that running, perhaps because it is our most basic solitary survival activity, produces the non-self-critical state more effectively than any other practice. He recommends running to everyone, from the weakest to the strongest. He feels that once an individual can run an hour without fatigue, it is almost certain that he or she will achieve the positive addiction state on a regular basis.

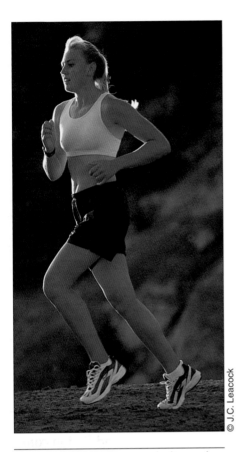

© J.C. Leacock

Is it possible to be too dedicated to activity, fitness, or training?

If competition is avoided and the runner runs alone in a pleasant setting, addiction should occur within the year.

I knew I was addicted to running long before Dr. Glasser wrote his book; it took far less than an hour per day of running or a year to achieve. Over the years the addiction to running has evolved to an addiction to activity. It works with hiking, cycling, cross-country skiing, swimming, even weight training, so long as I keep it noncompetitive and uncritical. As interests change or injuries occur, I've been able to transfer the addiction to new activities. And the addiction ensures that I will remain active for the rest of my life.

Is it possible to be too dedicated to activity, fitness, or training—to be negatively addicted or dependent? Probably so. An old friend, the eminent and venerable sport psychologist Dr. William Morgan, first called attention to the possibility, noting runners who were so addicted that they neglected family and work. Some continued to train in spite of an illness or injury (Morgan 1979). I too have seen runners with an obsessive compulsion for their sport. On closer inspection it seemed that some lives were confounded with other problems, that these people had turned to running as therapy. Several studies have linked compulsive running with the eating disorder anorexia nervosa. Others, however, found that addicted runners fell within the normal range of behavior whereas anorexics did not.

For my part I'd prefer a negative addiction to running over an addiction to alcohol or drugs. The compulsive activity may alter family relationships and work performance, but so does alcohol or drug abuse, and running won't destroy the body and the mind. The obsession with running may serve as a therapy, just as activity has served to reduce anxiety and depression. I've long thought that it might be possible to substitute a positive for a negative addiction, that a commitment to exercise might help a smoker give up the habit. Though this clearly works for some individuals, its application is limited by the sizable dropout rates common to exercise and smoking cessation programs.

Summary

Health has been called "the first of all liberties." What some call optimal health or wellness implies a vitality and zest for living that is much more than the absence of disease. Our definition of health also embraces psychological, emotional, or mental health. Thus, healthy people are free from disease, anxiety, and depression; their physical condition, nutritional state, and emotional outlook enable them to carry out daily tasks with vigor and alertness, without undue fatigue, and with ample energy to enjoy leisure-time pursuits and meet unforeseen emergencies.

The International Society of Sport Psychology (Tenenbaum and Singer 1992) believes that the benefits of regular vigorous activity include

- reduced state anxiety,
- decreased level of mild to moderate depression,
- reductions in neuroticism and anxiety,
- an adjunct to professional treatment of severe depression,
- reduction of stress indices, and
- beneficial emotional effects for all ages and both sexes.

We have seen how regular moderate activity serves to enhance both physical and mental health. Now let's explore the role of health care in the active life.

3

Activity and Personal Health

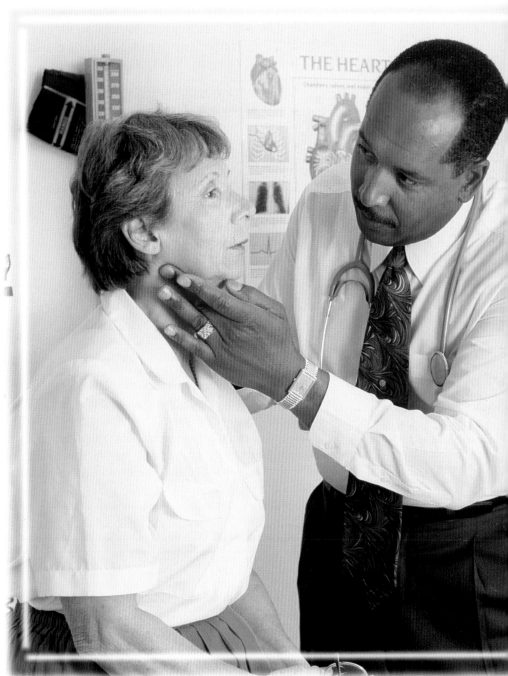

"Better to hunt
in fields, for
health unbought,
Than fee the
doctor for a
nauseous
draught.
The wise, for
cure, on exer-
cise depend:
God never made
his work for man
to mend."

John Dryden

The so-called American health care system is not about health, nor is it a system; instead it is a chaotic mixture of doctors, hospitals, drug and insurance companies, lawyers, and—oh, yes—patients, held together by market factors, mutual dependence, and self-interest. It is focused not on prevention or health, but on the treatment of illness, disease, and disabling injury. It isn't a system because it wasn't planned; it just grew. It defies economic theory; if demand goes down, prices go up. Worst of all, it has fostered an unhealthy attitude: If I ignore commonsense health habits and become sick or injured, the health care system will perform a miracle cure, and the insurance will pay the enormous costs. Insurance programs have insulated individuals from the real costs of treatment, thereby reducing incentives for good habits and cost containment. At the same time this so-called health care system leaves a staggering 44 million citizens without health insurance (up from 37 million in 1993)! Meaningful reform will require changes in all parts of the system.

- Doctors who gravitated toward specialization to enhance stature, income, and lifestyle and to fit a reimbursement system that paid for procedures will return to primary care, education, and prevention.
- Hospitals that became highly competitive corporate profit centers will return to cooperation and community service.
- Pharmaceutical corporations that invested millions to develop and billions to market new drugs will settle for a bit less on the bottom line.
- Insurance companies that practiced cherry picking, insuring only the healthy, will cover everyone, with fair rates and simplified forms.
- Lawyers who filed questionable malpractice cases for huge contingency fees will adjust to reasonable fees and tort reform.
- Patients who impatiently expected instant cures will assume greater responsibility for their health.
- Politicians who accepted massive contributions from all parties but patients will muster the courage to do the right thing.

Prevention is inexpensive; crisis medicine is not.

A carefully planned system will cover everyone; emphasize prevention and individual responsibility; charge more for bad habits (smoking, inactivity, not using a bicycle or motorcycle helmet); and limit the use of high-cost procedures, especially for the very old or terminally ill. Prevention is inexpensive; crisis medicine is not. The active life is the enlightened, responsible, and cost-effective way to disease prevention. It should be the keystone of a true health care system.

This chapter will help you

- recognize the values and limitations of health screening and early detection,
- develop a schedule for periodic medical examinations,
- determine the need for a pre-exercise medical exam, and
- understand the risks and benefits of regular moderate physical activity.

We're Number . . . 37?!

The World Health Organization's year 2000 ranking of national health care systems found that the United States spends more on health care per person ($3,724) than any other country, yet ranks 37th in overall health care quality. Why? One reason is that the United States fails to insure 44 million citizens amid a patchwork of private insurance and government programs. We spend billions on diagnostics, drugs, and procedures but little on prevention. Japan, which spends only $1,759 per person per year, beat the United States by four and a half years in the category of how long people live in good health, not just how long they live.

Many Americans have come to rely on their doctors to take care of their health. Of course, it doesn't work; your doctor can't make you stop smoking, lose weight, eat less fat, fasten your seat belt, or get regular exercise. These simple habits have more to do with health and disease than all the influences of medicine. More than half of all disease and death can be attributed to lifestyle. Granted, medical tests and treatments that prevent or minimize disease and disability are available, but not all of the procedures require a physician. Let's review features and limitations of health screening, early diagnosis, and the medical examination.

Health Screening

I have the pleasure of working in two bureaucracies, a university and a federal agency. Though they are different in many respects, they share an interest in the health of their employees: Both have employee health or wellness programs. Most wellness programs utilize a computerized health risk analysis as the start of a comprehensive health screening program. The analysis uses answers to questions about health habits and some basic information (age, sex, weight, blood pressure, cholesterol) to calculate health risks and to compute one's risk age. An overweight smoker with a family history of heart disease may have a risk age years above his or her chronological age. The health risk analysis is a simple, low-cost way to focus future health habits. A sample health risk analysis and longevity estimate are included in figures 3.6 and 3.7 (pages 63 through 67) at the end of this chapter.

Results from a cholesterol test could lead to a class on healthy food choices, an activity program, or even a doctor's visit and a prescription for cholesterol-lowering medication. The principle is simple: Use low-cost approaches to identify health habits and risks, apply more expensive tests but only for those at risk, and reserve high-cost tests and treatments for those in real need. Years ago, testing advocates thought health screening tests should be applied broadly. Now we realize that many tests should be reserved for those who, by virtue of age, risk factors, family history, or symptoms, are most in need of the procedure. Generalized testing is costly, wastes the time and effort of medical personnel, and risks false positive results (indication of a problem when none exists).

Various factors, including age, sex, health risks, family history, and occupation, influence the need for health screening. Young, apparently healthy individuals do well with infrequent tests, unless, of course, they have a family history or symptoms or they change habits. Regrettably, age alone increases the need for certain onerous tests, such as a colonoscope (for colon cancer) and digital prostate examination. A family history of glaucoma raises the need for a regular glaucoma test, and occupational exposure to noise or toxic chemicals calls for evaluation of hearing or lung function, respectively. A comprehensive worksite wellness program provides a wide range of health screening procedures (see figure 3.1), along with appropriate immunizations (e.g., flu shots for retired employees) and booster shots.

Early Detection

For a time there was great interest in the development of tests to detect problems such as cancer. The idea was that early detection would improve the prognosis for

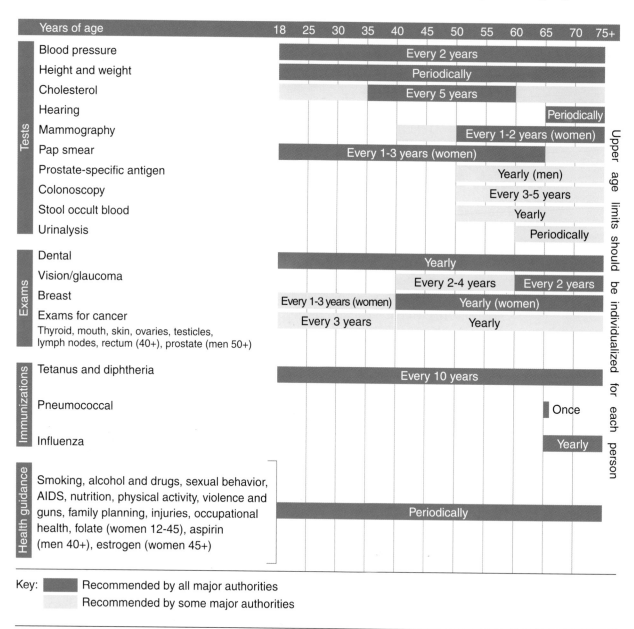

Figure 3.1 Adult preventive care timeline: recommendations of major authorities.

Early detection is meaningless if there is no effective treatment for the disease.

recovery. Indeed, some studies showed that early detection was associated with extended survival. Fine, so long as the extension of life exceeds the improvement in detection time. Early detection is meaningless, however, if there is no effective treatment for the disease. Of course, if the disease can be transmitted (e.g., AIDS) and one can effectively limit its spread, early detection makes sense from a public health standpoint.

In recent years medical opinion has changed concerning the course of treatment for several problems. For example, in older men, aggressive treatment of prostate cancer (surgery, radiation) has not proven superior to benign neglect. Survival time doesn't improve and the quality of life is often impaired. Back operations and heart surgery, even for patients with obvious symptoms, have been performed more often than necessary, leading one to question the accuracy of detection and diagnosis. But many tests are warranted, especially when they lead to changes in behaviors. Low-cost blood pressure and cholesterol tests can identify problems while there is still time to slow, stop, or even reverse the disease process. So if your age, sex, race, family history, health habits, or exposures put you at risk for a disease, by all means utilize an early detection test, as long as the proposed test meets the following criteria:

- The disease has a significant effect on the quality of life.
- Acceptable methods of treatment are available.
- Treatment during the asymptomatic (no symptom) period significantly reduces disability or death.
- Early treatment yields a superior result.
- Detection tests are available at a reasonable cost.
- The incidence of the disease in the population is sufficient to justify the cost of screening.

Few tests meet these criteria; blood pressure tests, breast examinations, and Pap smears do, whereas exercise stress tests, diabetes screening, and X-rays for lung cancer do not. Surprisingly, the routine (annual) medical examination also fails to meet the criteria.

Blood Pressure

High blood pressure, or hypertension, a silent killer with no obvious symptoms, is easy and inexpensive to test. Moreover, several acceptable methods of treatment are available, and successful control extends the quantity and quality of life. Systolic pressure is the pressure exerted against arterial walls when the heart contracts to send blood into the system. Diastolic pressure is the pressure against arterial walls between beats, when the heart is relaxed. Both measures contribute to the mean arterial pressure, and both have consequences for your health. Use the information in table 3.1 to evaluate your blood pressure.

Borderline and stage 1 cases often respond to diet, weight loss, and exercise. Stage 2 cases that remain elevated with diet, weight loss, exercise, and stress reduction will also require medication, as will most stage 3 and stage 4 cases. Studies clearly show the value of controlling blood pressure.

Aerobic exercise combined with weight loss is recommended for the management of elevated blood pressure in sedentary, overweight individuals (Blumenthal et al. 2000). High blood pressure can damage arterial walls and contribute to atherosclerosis, and excess pressure increases the risk of strokes. Though salt intake, being overweight, and stress may exacerbate the problem, the cause is poorly understood, and more than 90 percent of all cases are of unknown origin. Modern molecular biology will someday unlock the cause of these constricted arteries, but you can't wait for someday. Check your pressure regularly, and never rely on a single measure. If the pressure is elevated in several checks, restrict salt and fat, lose weight, engage in regular moderate activity, and learn how to manage stress. If all that isn't enough, or if the pressure is above 160, see your physician. New medications provide control of blood pressure with fewer side effects. But don't rely on medications for control; continue with diet, exercise, weight loss, and stress management.

Table 3.1 Blood Pressure Evaluation			
	Systolic BP	**Diastolic BP**	**Action**
Normal BP	<130 mm Hg	<85 mm Hg	Retest annually
Borderline	130-139	85-89	Retest in 6 mo
Hypertension			
Stage 1	140-159	90-99	Recheck
Stage 2	160-179	100-109	See doctor soon*
Stage 3	180-210	110-120	See doctor very soon
Stage 4	>210	>120	See doctor now!

*For recheck, diet, weight loss, activity, stress reduction, and possible medication.

Medical Examination

The typical medical examination includes a history, physical examination, and tests dictated by the patient's age and sex and the outcome of the exam. In the past, we all assumed that the annual medical examination would help us stay healthy and reduce the likelihood of illness or premature death. But when researchers compared those who had annual exams with those who did not, they found an equal number of chronic diseases and deaths in both groups. Today many doctors agree that for persons with no symptoms or chronic disease, the annual medical exam is a waste of time and money. A past president of the American Medical Association has said he hasn't had a routine physical since he joined the army decades ago, and he asks patients who request a check-up, "What do you want one for?" Let's consider a typical scenario to see why the annual medical exam pays off for the doctor and the laboratory but not for the patient.

Joe is a typical patient; he is 45, somewhat overweight and out of shape, smokes a pack a day, and indulges his love for meat and potatoes. His company pays for his annual medical exam, so the physician schedules a battery of tests, lowers the actual workload and invalidates the prediction of fitness and work capacity.

The stress test should be terminated when the subject cannot continue or has symptoms of exertional intolerance (chest pain, intolerable fatigue) or distress (staggering, dizziness, confusion, pallor, labored breathing, or nausea), when there are significant electrocardiographic changes, or when blood pressure drops in spite of an increasing workload. Termination of the test at some predetermined percentage of the assumed maximal heart rate, on the other hand, risks missing important signs or symptoms. As I have noted, the maximal heart rate is highly variable. Using an age-related maximal heart rate (e.g., 220 beats per minute minus age equals the predicted maximal heart rate) can lead to substantial errors. For example, the maximal heart rate for 40-year-old patients may average 180 beats per minute (bpm) (220 minus 40 equals 180), but the range goes from below144 to above 216. So a test terminated at 85 percent of the predicted maximal heart rate (.85 times 180 equals 153 bpm) may be too strenuous for a few and much too easy for others.

Maximal Heart Rate

The variability in maximal heart rate, as defined by a statistic called the standard deviation (SD), is plus or minus 12 bpm: 68 percent of all cases fall within plus or minus one SD, 95 percent within plus or minus two SD, and 99 percent within plus or minus three SD. So, for our example, it is likely that one in a hundred 40-year-olds may have a maximal heart rate below 144 or above 216. Incidentally, as you'll see in chapter 4, this variability in maximal heart rate complicates the use of the heart rate for the prescription of exercise. And to make matters more confusing, the standard deviation for maximal heart rate goes up to 15 bpm for older individuals!

The Exercise Electrocardiogram

The electrocardiogram (ECG) is a strip of paper with a record of the heart's electrical activity. Each complete ECG cycle (see figure 3.3) represents one beat of the heart. The P wave shows the electrical activity that immediately precedes the contraction of the upper chambers, or atria. The QRS complex represents the electrical discharge of the lower chambers, or ventricles, and the T wave results when the depolarized ventricles are recharged. Under normal conditions the heart receives excitation at the sinoatrial node, via the sympathetic nervous system. The impulse spreads across the atria, causing contraction of the upper chambers as the impulse flows, and finally arrives at the atrioventricular node. Here the impulse finds its way down specialized fibers to the muscle of the ventricles, causing them to contract and pump blood to the body.

The ECG is wired to indicate a positive deflection when the depolarization wave is flowing toward the positive electrode. The P wave and QRS complex normally yield positive deflections. If the stimulus to contract originates from the wrong direction (e.g., from the ventricles), the QRS could deflect downward. Because the recording paper moves at a specified speed (usually 25 millimeters per second), the width of the wave can provide information about the rate of conduction. For example, if conduction is slow or blocked, the base of the QRS will be broad. The physician, nurse, or exercise test technologist administering a stress

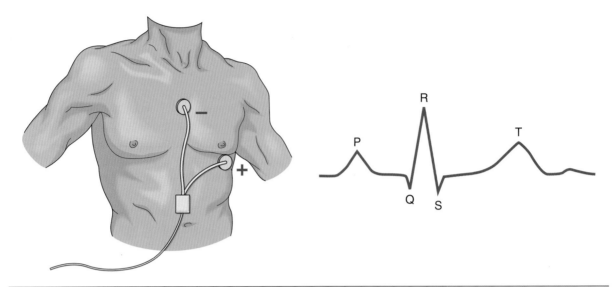

Figure 3.3 The ECG cycle. *P* wave indicates depolarization of atria. *QRS* wave is caused by spread of excitation through ventricles. *T* wave indicates repolarization of ventricles.

test pays careful attention to the ECG waveform as it travels across the screen of the oscilloscope. Changes of sufficient importance to terminate the test include the following:

- S-T segment depression in excess of 0.2 millivolts (mv) (2 millimeters below baseline)

- Irregular rhythms (e.g., premature ventricular contractions, or PVCs), particularly when they originate in the ventricles and come in volleys of 3 or more or as many as 10 per minute

- Left ventricular conduction disturbances

Exercise-induced PVCs may lead to ventricular tachycardia (extremely rapid rate) and occasionally to fibrillation, an uncontrolled and uncoordinated action of heart muscle fibers that is incapable of pumping blood. Fibrillation requires immediate emergency action: The defibrillator provides a strong direct current that depolarizes the entire heart muscle, thereby allowing return to the normal pattern of stimulation. Conduction disturbances occasionally occur during stress tests, so it is important to have emergency equipment and trained personnel available when high-risk patients are being evaluated. Fortunately, most patients recover and are able to return to supervised activity after defibrillation. Tests conducted on apparently healthy individuals are not considered unsafe, but test administrators should be thoroughly trained in cardiopulmonary resuscitation (CPR) and other emergency techniques.

Test Results

When the exercise stress test results are suggestive of heart problems (e.g., ECG abnormalities, chest pain, or abnormal blood pressure response) the test is called positive. Stress test findings are verified when they are confirmed with cardiac catheterization, an invasive imaging technique. In this procedure a catheter is inserted into a blood vessel in the leg and worked into position in the aorta. An opaque dye is injected into each coronary artery to allow X-ray detection of narrowing due to atherosclerosis. Results of a positive stress test are considered

People With Disabilities

Each disability carries its own restrictions, but each has potential as well. People with disabilities participate and compete all the way up to international competitions, but only after establishing control over their conditions. They have learned to ski, to kayak, to do just about anything, and more opportunities are becoming available. Wheelchair athletes compete in marathons, play basketball, and fish at special access sites. Individuals with multiple sclerosis respond better to moderate activity, such as swimming. For more information contact your recreation department or community service organizations.

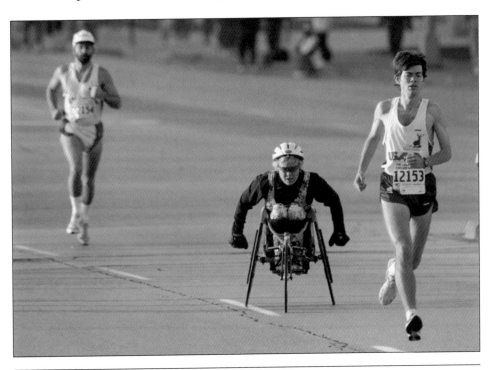

A disability needn't prevent you from living the active life.

Racial Considerations

A series of articles documented the greater prevalence of hypertension among African Americans (Lubell 1988). One in every three African-American adults has hypertension, compared with one in four non-African Americans, and African Americans are two times more likely to have moderate hypertension and three times more likely to have severe hypertension than whites. Although African Americans will benefit from aerobic and moderate lifting activities, those with hypertension may want to avoid very heavy lifting or exercises with an isometric (static) component, since straining against a heavy load can elevate blood pressure dramatically. Aerobic exercise and weight loss will help lower blood pressure, but people with hypertension should undergo a pre-exercise medical examination, follow dietary recommendations, and take prescribed medications.

Health and Wellness

In the past health was defined as the absence of disease, and that is how many individuals still think of the term. Recently the definition of health has been expanded to include a state of complete physical, mental, and emotional well-being, not merely the absence of disease or infirmity. In that context the relationship of activity to health becomes clearer. The relationship of health and wellness is equally clear. Ardell (1984) defined wellness as "a conscious and deliberate approach to an advanced state of physical and psychological/spiritual health." So wellness defines movement toward an advanced state of health, which is also called optimal or high-level health (figure 3.5).

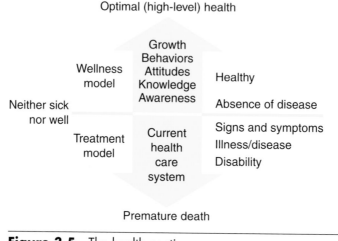

Figure 3.5 The health continuum.

The old view of health placed illness on one side of a line and health on the other, with doctors and the treatment-oriented health care system defending the line. Wellness, on the other hand, is viewed as a dynamic process where you—the individual—are responsible for your health. The health care system is treatment-oriented: Workers in the system focus on correcting problems brought on by illness, disease, injury, or disability. Wellness involves disease prevention and promoting behaviors that lower the risk of illness or injury. The treatment system employs an army of high-priced professionals and costs billions of dollars. Wellness relies on individual responsibility, low-cost helpers, and reduced reliance on costly specialists and procedures. The active life is the keystone of health and wellness.

Health Risk Analysis

Use the health risk analysis in figure 3.6 as a learning tool to identify positive and negative aspects of your health behavior. Though many of the effects are based on real findings from large epidemiological investigations, the estimates are generalized and should not be taken too literally. It is impossible to predict with accuracy how long you will live or when you will die. A more accurate estimate can be achieved by estimating risk according to age, sex, and race, using computerized analyses.

Plus one (+1) represents a positive effect that could add a year to your life or life to your years, and minus one (–1) indicates a loss in the quantity or quality of life. Complete each section and record the totals in figure 3.7 on page 67.

Coronary Heart Disease (CHD) Risk Factors

Cholesterol, total cholesterol/HDL ratio

under 160	160-200	200-220	220-240	over 240	
<3	3-4	4-5	5-6	>6	
+2	+1	−1	−2	−4	_____

Blood pressure $\left(\frac{systolic}{diastolic}\right)$

110	110-130	130-150	150-170	170	
60-80	60-80	80-90	90-100	>100	
+1	0	−1	−2	−4	_____

Smoking

never	quit	smoke cigar or pipe or close family member smokes	1 pack cigarettes daily	2 or more packs daily	
+1	0	−1	−3	−5	_____

Heredity

no family history of CHD	1 close relative over 60 with CHD	2 close relatives over 60 with CHD	1 close relative under 60 with CHD	2 or more close relatives under 60 with CHD	
+2	0	−1	−2	−4	_____

Body weight (or fat)

5 lb below desirable weight (<10% fat—M; <16% fat—F)	5 lb below to 4 lb above desirable weight (10-15% fat—M; 16-22% fat—F)	5-20 lb overweight (15-20% fat—M; 22-30% fat—F)	20-35 lb overweight (20-25% fat—M; 30-35% fat—F)	>35 lb overweight (>25% fat—M; >35% fat—F)	
+2	+1	0	−2	−3	_____

Sex

female under 55 years	female over 55 years	male	stocky male	bald, stocky male	
0	−1	−1	−2	−4	_____

Stress

phlegmatic, unhurried, generally happy	ambitious but generally relaxed	sometimes hard-driving, time-competitive	hard-driving, time-conscious, competitive (Type A)	Type A with repressed hostility	
+1	0	0	−1	−3	_____

Physical activity

high-intesity, over 30 minutes daily	intermittent, 20-30 minutes 3-5 times/week	moderate, 10-20 minutes 3-5 times/week	light, 10-20 minutes 1-2 times/week	little or none	
+2	+2	+1	0	−2	_____

Total: I CHD Risk Factors _____

Enter on figure 3.7

(continued)

Figure 3.6 Health risk summary.

II Health Habits (related to good health and longevity)

Breakfast

daily	sometimes	none	coffee	coffee and doughnut	
+1	0	−1	−2	−3	_____

Regular meals

3 or more	2 daily	not regular	fad diets	starve and stuff	
+1	0	−1	−2	−3	_____

Sleep

7-8 hr	8-9 hr	6-7 hr	9 hr	6 hr	
+1	0	0	−1	−2	_____

Alcohol

none	women 3/wk	men 1-2 daily	2-6 daily	6 daily	
+1	+1	+1	−2	−4	_____

Total: II Health Habits　_____

Enter on figure 3.7

III Medical Factors

Medical exam and screening tests (blood pressure, diabetes, glaucoma)

regular tests, see doctor when necessary	periodic medical exam and selected tests	periodic medical exam	sometimes get tests	no tests or medical exams	
+1	+1	0	0	−1	_____

Heart

no history of problems self or family	some history	rheumatic fever as child, no murmur now	rheumatic fever as child, have murmur	have ECG abnormality and/or angina pectoris	
+1	0	−1	−2	−3	_____

Lung (including pneumonia and tuberculosis)

no problem	some past problem	mild asthma or bronchitis	emphysema, severe asthma, or bronchitis	severe lung problems	
+1	0	−1	−2	−3	_____

Digestive tract

no problem	occasional diarrhea, loss of appetite	frequent diarrhea or stomach upset	ulcers, colitis, gall bladder, or liver problems	severe gastrointestinal disorders	
+1	0	−1	−2	−3	_____

Diabetes

no problem or family history	controlled hypoglycemia (low blood sugar)	hypoglycemia and family history	mild diabetes (diet and exercise)	diabetes (insulin)	
+1	0	−1	−2	−3	_____

Drugs

seldom take	minimal but regular use of aspirin or other drugs	heavy use of aspirin or other drugs	regular use of amphetamines, barbiturates, or psychogenic drugs	heavy use of amphetamines, barbiturates, or psychogenic drugs	
+1	0	−1	−2	−3	_____

Total: III Medical Factors　_____

Enter on figure 3.7

Figure 3.6　*(continued)*

Drugs

seldom take	minimal but regular use of aspirin or other drugs	heavy use of aspirin or other drugs	regular use of amphet-amines, barbitu-rates, or psychogenic drugs	heavy use of amphetamines, barbiturates, or psychogenic drugs	
+1	0	−1	−2	−3	_____

Total: III Medical Factors _____

Enter on figure 3.7

IV Safety Factors

Driving in car

4,000 mi/ year, mostly local	4,000-6,000 mi/ year, local and some highway	6,000-8,000 mi/ year, local and highway	8,000-10,000 mi/ year, highway and some local	10,000 mi/ year, mostly highway	
+1	0	0	−1	−2	_____

Using seat belts

always	most of time (75%)	on highway only	seldom (25%)	never	
+1	0	−1	−2	−3	_____

Risk-taking behavior

(motorcycle, skydive, mountain climb, fly small plane, etc.)

some with careful preparation	never	occasional	often	try anything for thrills	
+1	0	−1	−1	−2	_____

Total: IV Safety Factors _____

Enter on figure 3.7

V Personal Factors

Diet

low-fat, high-complex carbohydrates	balanced, moderate fat	balanced, typical fat	fad diets	starve and stuff	
+2	+1	0	−1	−2	_____

Longevity

grandparents lived past 90, parents past 80	grandparents lived past 80, parents past 70	grandparents lived past 70, parents past 60	few relatives lived past 60	few relatives lived past 50	
+2	+1	0	−1	−3	_____

Love and marriage

happily married	married	unmarried	divorced	extramarital relationship	
+2	+1	0	−1	−3	_____

Education

postgraduate or master craftsman	college graduate or skilled craftsman	some college or trade school	high school graduate	grade school graduate	
+1	+1	0	−1	−2	_____

Job satisfaction

enjoy job, see results, room for advancement	enjoy job, see some results, able to advance	job OK, no results, nowhere to go	dislike job	hate job	
+1	+1	0	−1	−2	_____

(continued)

Figure 3.6 (continued)

V Personal Factors (continued)

Social

| have some close friends +1 | have some friends 0 | have no good friends −1 | stuck with people I don't enjoy −2 | have no friends at all −3 | _____ |

Race

| white or Asian 0 | black or Hispanic −1 | American Indian −2 | | | _____ |

Total: V Personal Factors _____

Enter on figure 3.7

VI Psychological Factors

Outlook

| feel good about present and future +1 | satisfied 0 | unsure about present or future −1 | unhappy in present, don't look forward to future −2 | miserable, rather not get out of bed −3 | _____ |

Depression

| no family history of depression +1 | some family history—I feel OK 0 | family history and I am mildly depressed −1 | sometimes feel life isn't worth living −2 | thoughts of suicide −3 | _____ |

Anxiety

| seldom anxious +1 | occasionally anxious 0 | often anxious −1 | always anxious −2 | panic attacks −3 | _____ |

Relaxation

| relax meditate daily +1 | relax often 0 | seldom relax −1 | usually tense −2 | always tense −3 | _____ |

Total: VI Psychological Factors _____

Enter on figure 3.7

VII For Women Only

Health care

| regular breast and Pap exam +1 | occasional breast and Pap exam 0 | never have exam −1 | treated disorder −2 | untreated cancer −4 | _____ |

Birth control pill

| never used +1 | quit 5 years ago 0 | still use, under 30 years 0 | use pill and smoke −2 | use pill, smoke, over 35 −3 | _____ |

Total: VII For Women Only _____

Enter on figure 3.7

Figure 3.6 (continued)

Category	Score (+/- years)			Life expectancy	
				Nearest age	Expectancy
I. CHD risk factors	☐			30	74
II. Health habits	☐			35	74
III. Medical factors	☐			40	75
IV. Safety factors	☐			45	76
V. Personal factors	☐			50	76
VI. Psychological factors	☐			55	77
VII. For women only	☐ + ☐ = ☐			60	78
	Total Your Longevity			65	80
	age estimate			70	82

Figure 3.7 Health risk summary. Now go back and see how you can add years to your life by improving behaviors and lifestyle. Check each category for possible changes you would like to make in your current lifestyle.

What Can You Do?

If you find that your risk of heart disease is high, there are a number of steps you can take to lower the risk, including the following:

- Engage in regular moderate physical activity.
- Eat less saturated fat and more fresh fruits and vegetables.
- Eat soy protein and olive oil.
- Keep your body mass index below 25 (see page 263).
- Take an aspirin daily or every other (e/o) day.
- Take daily supplements of vitamin E and folic acid.
- Have one alcoholic drink (red wine or beer) daily or e/o day.

In subsequent chapters I will tell you the reasons that you should consider these and other steps.

Summary

Until recently the medical community has been cautious concerning exercise, suggesting a visit to the physician and even a stress test before participation. This is understandable given that few medical schools offer more than one or two lectures on exercise physiology. Unless your doctor is active or has special training in physiology or sports medicine, he or she may know very little about the benefits of activity and how to prescribe exercise to achieve those benefits. But as the benefits and risks become better understood, physicians are turning to exercise physiologists to design and conduct preventive and rehabilitative exercise programs.

Of course, you don't have to see your physician in order to participate in moderate activity such as walking. If you feel good and answer no to all the questions in the Par-Q questionnaire (page 53), you don't have to spend hundreds of dollars to confirm what you already know. Start slowly, increase intensity and duration gradually, and read the next section of this book. And use health screening, early detection, and periodic medical examinations to help you maintain your health.

PART II
Aerobic Fitness

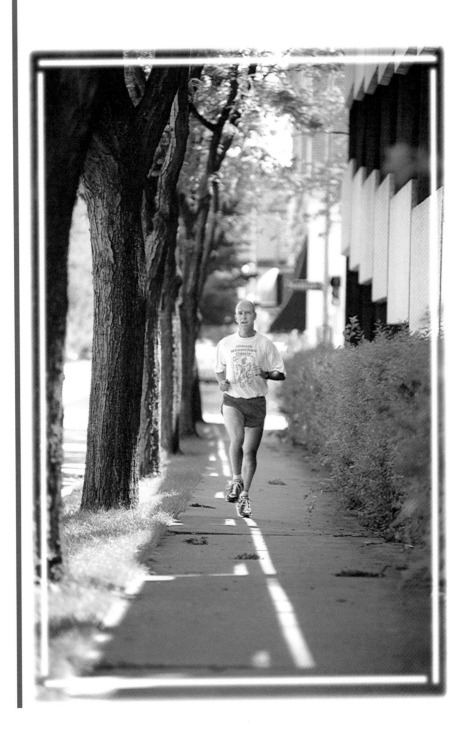

Somewhere above the pace of your normal daily activities but well below maximal effort you will find aerobic exercise. If you do aerobic exercise often enough you will improve your aerobic fitness, and as fitness improves you'll further enhance your health, appearance, vitality, and quality of life. Aerobic fitness describes how well you are able to take oxygen from the atmosphere into the lungs and then the blood and pump it via the heart and circulatory system to working muscles where it is utilized to oxidize carbohydrate and fat to produce energy. No other measure says more about the health and capacity of your lungs, heart, circulatory system, and, most important, your skeletal muscles.

Rhythmic large-muscle activities such as brisk walking, jogging, cycling, swimming, cross-country skiing, and rowing are aerobic exercises. They demand sustained increases in respiration, circulation, and muscle metabolism and lead to adaptations in the systems and muscles involved. Aerobic exercise is associated with health and longevity, regular participation in aerobic exercise improves aerobic fitness, and improved fitness further enhances health. In many physical, psychological, and social ways, aerobic fitness is good for health and the quality of life. It improves appearance, boosts self-confidence and body image, and opens the door to a challenging new world filled with new experiences and interesting people. Let's see how you can integrate fitness into your busy schedule so you can reap the many extra benefits.

4

Understanding Aerobic Fitness

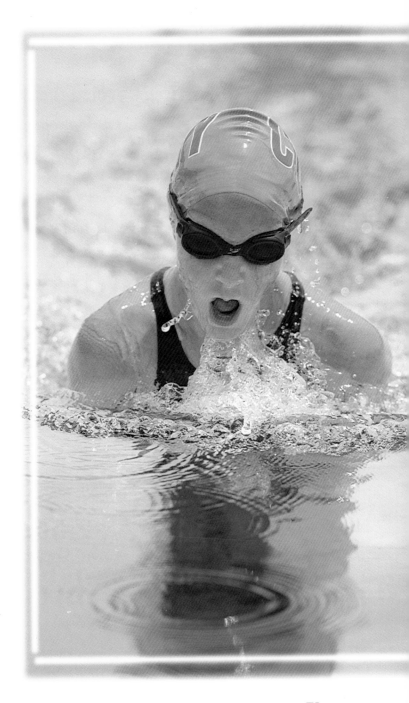

"The firm, the enduring, the simple, and the modest are near to virtue."

Confucius

To me, aerobic fitness is synonymous with endurance or stamina. It describes the ability, part inherited and part trained, to persevere or persist in strenuous or prolonged endeavors. Those who pursue fitness earn far more than enhanced health and performance. For many the process becomes more important than the goal, providing discipline, challenge, and time for reflection. For the moment we'll consider the physiology of fitness; later we'll ponder its other dimensions.

■ This chapter will help you

- understand the terms *aerobic* and *anaerobic*,
- determine the meaning of aerobic exercise and aerobic fitness,
- identify and experience the concept of anaerobic threshold, and
- understand the factors that influence aerobic fitness.

Aerobic Exercise

Dress for exercise, warm up, and head out at a walking pace. Increase the pace a little as each minute passes, going from a slow to a fast walk. At about five miles (8 kilometers) per hour (12 minutes per mile) you'll begin to jog. Continue to gradually increase your speed until the effort becomes uncomfortable, breathing becomes labored, and you doubt your ability to continue. Up to this point the exercise has been aerobic, which means "in the presence of oxygen." Energy has come from the oxidation of fat and carbohydrate. If you continued to increase the intensity of exercise, the muscles would make a transition to anaerobic, or nonoxidative, energy production, which involves intense effort of necessarily short duration and the accumulation of lactic acid in the muscles and blood.

Lactic acid is both an energy carrier and a metabolic by-product of intense effort. Its accumulation is a sign that you are using energy faster than it can be produced aerobically. Too much lactic acid interferes with the muscle's contractile and metabolic capabilities. Lactic acid and the high levels of carbon dioxide produced in vigorous effort are associated with labored breathing, fatigue, and discomfort. Aerobic exercise can be defined as exercise below the point at which blood lactic acid levels rise—the lactate threshold (see figure 4.1).

Fiber Types

Humans have three main types of muscle fibers: slow-twitch (slow oxidative, or SO) fibers that are efficient in the use of oxygen; a faster-contracting type that can work with oxygen or without (fast oxidative glycolytic, or FOG); and a fast-twitch fiber that uses muscle glycogen for short, intense contractions (fast glycolytic, or FG). As we go from a walk to a jog to a run we recruit SO, FOG, then FG fibers to help us go faster. Recruit too many FG fibers and the effort becomes anaerobic; the fibers produce lactic acid, and we are forced to slow down or stop (see figure 4.1).

Aerobic metabolism is far more efficient than anaerobic, yielding 38 molecules of adenosine triphosphate (ATP), the high-energy compound that fuels muscular contractions, per molecule of glucose, versus only 2 molecules of ATP via anaerobic metabolism. Because it produces little lactic acid, aerobic exercise is

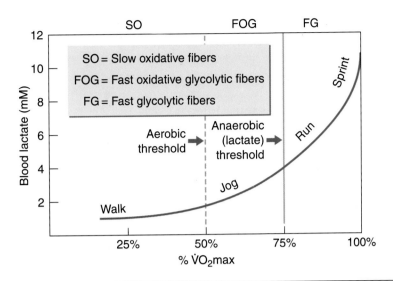

Figure 4.1 Anaerobic (lactate) threshold. As exercise intensity (percent $\dot{V}O_2$max) increases we recruit FOG fibers, then FG fibers. More blood lactate accumulates because FG fibers produce more lactic acid and because most muscle fibers are active and therefore unable to remove (take up) lactate.

The oxidation of abundant fat reserves during aerobic exercise ensures an adequate supply of energy for extended periods of effort.

relatively pleasant and relaxing, not painful. And the oxidation of abundant fat reserves during aerobic exercise ensures an adequate supply of energy for extended periods of effort. Aerobic exercise can be sustained for several minutes to many hours. You can carry on a conversation during moderate aerobic exercise.

Endurance

A biologist friend who has studied locomotion throughout the animal kingdom has noted that when it comes to running short distances, humans are inferior to other species. Cheetahs, gazelles, antelopes, horses, camels, even grizzly bears are much faster than humans. But as the distance increases, the human becomes more competitive, and at long distances, human endurance qualities stand out. Unfortunately, this superiority emerges only at distances few are willing to negotiate. When a proud Montana horseman bragged about the endurance and speed of his Arabian, a local physician wagered he could outrun the horse over a mountainous marathon course (26.2 miles, or 42.2 kilometers). Perhaps the distance wasn't long enough, because the horse finished 16 minutes ahead of the physician. Of course, it is also possible that the fit but 49-year-old physician was slightly past his prime, whereas the horse was not.

We have ample evidence that humans are able to cover 100 miles (161 kilometers) or more. The Tarahumara Indians of Mexico run more than 100 miles while kicking a small ball, and runners throughout the world do 100-mile footraces, sometimes over difficult mountain terrain. Early in the 20th century, crowds flocked to big cities to watch six-day races, in which athletes attempted to run as far as possible. Today the six-day record is well over 635 miles (1,022 kilometers), for an average of 106 miles (171 kilometers) per day! In spite of the publicity given short races and sports that emphasize bursts of speed, the human body has evolved with the capacity to accomplish prodigious feats of endurance.

Aerobic and anaerobic exercises differ in intensity; light to moderate activity is aerobic, whereas extremely vigorous or intense effort is anaerobic. Table 4.1 illustrates how heart rate and breathing increase with exercise intensity, and how we switch from burning fat to carbohydrate as exercise becomes more vigorous. The table also shows how the nervous system recruits different muscle fiber types as the effort becomes more intense.

Table 4.1　Levels of Exercise Intensity

| | | Exercise intensity | |
	Light	Moderate	Intense
Example exercise	Walking	Jogging	Running
Metabolism	Aerobic	Aerobic	Aerobic/anaerobic
Energy source	Fat and CHO	CHO and fat	CHO and fat
Heart rate	<120	120-150	>150
Breathing	Easy	Can talk easily	Hard to talk
Muscle fiber recruited	SO	FOG	FG

CHO = carbohydrate

Aerobic Fitness

Aerobic fitness, defined as the maximal capacity to take in, transport, and utilize oxygen, is best measured in a laboratory test called the maximal oxygen intake (or $\dot{V}O_2$max) test. The test, which defines the highest sustainable intensity of effort, requires a treadmill or other exercise device; a metabolic measurement system to measure oxygen, carbon dioxide, and the volume of expired air; and a computer to do the calculations. After a health risk assessment, the person being tested signs an informed consent form and is fitted with ECG electrodes to monitor the heart and measure heart rate.

After a brief warm-up, the individual begins the test wearing a mask or mouthpiece to direct the expired air into the analyzer. The test involves a walk (or run, for the more fit) on the treadmill, which is programmed to increase grade every minute or two. Oxygen intake is computed each minute as the test proceeds toward maximal effort. The test is terminated when the oxygen intake levels off in spite of increased treadmill grade, or when the individual can no longer keep up with the treadmill. The highest level of oxygen attained is called the maximal oxygen intake, or aerobic fitness.

$\dot{V}O_2$max Test

The $\dot{V}O_2$max test protocol, the result of many years of experience, is suitable for a wide range of individuals, from the sedentary to elite athletes. The test, which takes from 8 to 12 minutes, can utilize either metabolic measurements to measure oxygen intake or a table to estimate the value. The protocol allows the test to be tailored to the subject's level of fitness and previous training. Figure 4.2 describes the protocol, and table 4.2 provides information for the estimation of the $\dot{V}O_2$max. The individual being tested should not be allowed to hold on to the railing of the

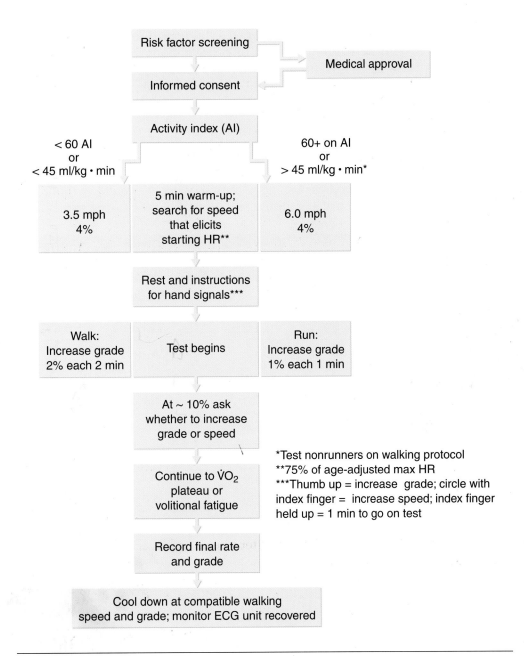

Figure 4.2 Flowchart for $\dot{V}O_2$max test protocol.

treadmill if the intention is to estimate the maximal value. Holding on to the railing reduces the workload and overestimates the estimation of oxygen uptake.

Use the final rate and grade on the treadmill to estimate the $\dot{V}O_2$max (see table 4.2). For example, if the last minute of the test was at 6 miles (9.7 kilometers) per hour and 10 percent grade, the aerobic fitness estimate is 50 ml/kg · min, or 50 milliliters of oxygen per kilogram of body weight per minute.

Scores in the range of three to four liters of oxygen per minute (L/min) are common, and values of five to six liters have been reported for endurance athletes. When reported in L/min (called *aerobic capacity*), the score provides information about the total capacity of the cardiorespiratory systems and is a good predictor of endurance performance in non-weight-bearing sports (e.g., cycling). However, because this value is related to body size, larger individuals tend to have higher scores. To eliminate the influence of body size, the maximal oxygen intake score in liters is divided by the body weight in kilograms (one kilogram equals 2.2 pounds). In this example, maximal oxygen intake score is three liters, and body weight is 60 kilograms (132 pounds):

$$3 \text{ L/min} \div 60 \text{ kg} = 50 \text{ ml/kg} \cdot \text{min}$$

Table 4.3 indicates typical values of aerobic fitness.

The resulting value allows direct comparison of individuals regardless of body size. This measure, also known as *aerobic power*, is more related to endurance performance in running and other weight-bearing sports, and it is the preferred

Table 4.2 Estimating $\dot{V}O_2$max: Approximate Oxygen Intake Requirements for Final Rate/Grade Combinations*

| Miles per hour | Grade | | | | |
	8%	10%	12%	14%	15%
Walk					
3.0 (4.8 km)		26	30	34	
3.5 (5.6 km)		29	34	39	
4.0 (6.4 km)		32	38	44	(48)
Run					
6.0 (9.7 km)	(47)	50	53	56	
7.0 (11.3 km)		58	61	65	
8.0 (12.9 km)		66	70	74	

*ml/kg · min; varies with efficiency. (Numbers in parentheses represent $\dot{V}O_2$max in ml/kg · min.)

Table 4.3 Fitness Comparison

Subjects	Age	Men (ml/kg · min)	Women (ml/kg · min)
Untrained	18-22	45	39
Active	18-22	50	43
Trained	18-22	57	53
Elite	18-22	70	63
World class	18-22	80+	70+
Untrained	40-50	36	27
Active	40-50	46	39
Trained	40-50	52	44
Elite	40-50	60+	50+

way to express aerobic fitness. If two individuals have the same score in liters, which one is more fit? If one weighs 60 kilograms as in the preceding example and the other weighs 100 kilograms (220 pounds), likewise divide the score for the latter by the respective body weight:

$$3 \text{ L/min} \div 100 \text{ kg} = 30 \text{ ml/kg} \cdot \text{min}$$

In a footrace, the one with a score of 50 would be better able to take in, transport, and utilize oxygen in the working muscles than the one with the score of 30. The average young male (18 to 25 years old) scores 45 to 48 ml/kg · min, and the average female scores 39 to 41. Active men score in the 50s and 60s and similarly active women in the 40s and 50s. Male endurance athletes have been measured in the 80s, and top female athletes are not far behind with scores in the 70s (see table 4.3). Although average values decline with age, as much as 8 to 10 percent per decade in sedentary populations, regular activity cuts the rate of decline in half (4 to 5 percent per decade), and aerobic training can cut that rate in half (2 to 3 percent per decade).

Measures that reflect the oxidative capacity of muscle reflect exercise *duration*, or how long a vigorous effort can be sustained.

Until recently, the aerobic fitness score ($\dot{V}O_2$max) was viewed as the best measure of fitness and was believed to be correlated to health and related to performance in work and sport. Though all this is still true, other ways to measure fitness have begun to emerge, and some seem better correlated to endurance and to performance. The maximal oxygen intake, or $\dot{V}O_2$max, test, which uses the highest score attained, is a test of exercise *intensity,* best correlated to events lasting 5 to 15 minutes. Measures that reflect the oxidative capacity of muscle (e.g., the lactate threshold) reflect exercise *duration,* or how long a vigorous effort can be sustained. So the lactate threshold is a better indicator of performance in activities lasting from 30 minutes or more to 3 hours or more (Sharkey 1991). The aerobic threshold indicates the level of effort that can be sustained for many hours (see figure 4.1).

Lactate (Anaerobic) Threshold

When exercise becomes very intense, more energy is produced anaerobically, lactic acid begins to accumulate in the blood, and carbon dioxide production increases along with the rate and depth of breathing. The discomfort caused by lactic acid and the labored breathing are sure signs that you have stepped across the anaerobic threshold. The threshold defines the upper limit of sustainable aerobic exercise, and it is a good indicator of endurance performance. Physiologists discourage use of the term anaerobic threshold, however, because not all fibers may be anaerobic; lactate may be produced in one muscle fiber and used as an energy source in another. So I'll use the more specific term *lactate threshold* (LT) to define the upper limit of aerobic metabolism and transition to anaerobic metabolism.

Threshold measurements can be made during the $\dot{V}O_2$max test. Blood is drawn after each stage (percent grade) of the treadmill test and analyzed in a lactate analyzer. The lactate threshold may be defined as the point at which lactate production increases dramatically or at a particular level (e.g., four millimoles [mM]), and reported as a percent of the $\dot{V}O_2$max or the velocity at LT. A less invasive way to estimate the threshold involves measuring and plotting the rise in ventilation during the progressive treadmill test. The *ventilatory threshold* (VT) is defined as the point at which the ventilation (in liters of air per minute) rises disproportionally, a point that has been called breakaway ventilation. This rise in ventilation provides a perceptible signal that indicates you are flirting with exhaustion and had better ease off. Perceptive athletes learn to listen to the information their bodies provide. Finally, you can estimate your threshold with a field test.

Estimating the Threshold

The lactate threshold is a better indicator of endurance performance than aerobic fitness ($\dot{V}O_2$max) in events such as a 10-kilometer road race. The lactate threshold indicates the oxygen utilization capabilities of the muscles. You can predict your threshold using equations developed by Dr. Art Weltman (1989) at the University of Virginia.

The prediction equation uses the time for a 3,200-meter run to predict the lactate threshold, expressed as the $\dot{V}O_2$ (oxygen uptake) at the threshold (4 millimoles [mM] lactate). You can use this value and the results of your aerobic capacity test to determine the percentage of the maximum that you can sustain.

For men:

$$\dot{V}O_2 \text{ (ml/[kg} \cdot \text{min])} = 122.0 - (5.31 \times [3{,}200\text{-m time in min*}])$$

*In minutes and decimal fractions; e.g., 30 s = .5 min.

For women:

$$\dot{V}O_2 = (-1.123 \, [3{,}200\text{-m time}]) + 61.57$$

(note negative in equation)

Example:

A 40-year-old male with 3,200-meter time of 14 minutes:

$$\dot{V}O_2 = 122 - (5.31 \times 14)$$

$$= 122 - 74.34$$

$$= 47.66$$

Divide the result (47.66) by the max (56) to get the lactate threshold as a percentage of the max, $47.6 \div 56 = 85\%$ of the $\dot{V}O_2$max. Use the aerobic fitness and threshold tests to gauge the progress of your training.

Though the threshold measurements are often similar, they can be disassociated, indicating that they are measuring somewhat different aspects of the exercise response. Taken together, the $\dot{V}O_2$max and the lactate threshold tell a lot about aerobic fitness and performance potential, with the $\dot{V}O_2$max indicating the capacity for intensity and the threshold defining the capacity for duration or endurance. Now let us explore the factors that influence aerobic fitness.

Dimensions of Aerobic Fitness

There are three dimensions of aerobic fitness; all of them can be determined in a single treadmill test.

Test	Measures	Best related to
$\dot{V}O_2max$	Intensity	Events lasting 5 to 15 min (1 to 3 miles, or 1.6 to 4.8 kilometers)
Lactate threshold	Duration	Events over 15 minutes (10K to marathon)
Aerobic threshold*	Long duration	Prolonged work or sport (hours)

*Defined as the first rise, or breakpoint, in the lactate or ventilatory response to increasing rate or grade of exercise (see figure 4.1).

The aerobic threshold defines the level of effort that can be sustained for prolonged periods. Expressed as a percentage of $\dot{V}O_2max$, it may be low or high, depending on your level of activity. It can be increased via training according to the principles presented in chapter 6.

Factors Influencing Aerobic Fitness

Is a high aerobic fitness score the product of heredity or training? How do other factors such as sex, age, and body fat influence your attainable level of fitness?

Heredity

The way to become a world-class endurance athlete is to pick your parents carefully.

It takes tremendous natural endowment and years of systematic training to achieve high-level endurance performances. Canadian researchers have studied differences in aerobic fitness among fraternal (dizygotic) and identical (monozygotic) twins and found that intrapair differences were far greater among fraternal than among identical twins. The largest difference between identical twins was smaller than the smallest difference between fraternal pairs (Klissouras 1976). More recently, Bouchard et al. (1999) estimated that heredity accounts for 47 percent or more of the variance in $\dot{V}O_2max$ values, and Sundet, Magnus, and Tambs (1994) contend that more than half of the variance in maximal aerobic power is due to genotypic differences, with the remainder accounted for by environmental factors (nutrition, training). This supports the notion that the way to become a world-class endurance athlete is to pick your parents carefully, especially your mother, since maternal transmission accounts for almost 60 percent of the inherited component (Bouchard et al. 1999)!

We inherit many factors that are important to aerobic fitness, including the maximal capacity of the respiratory and cardiovascular systems, a larger heart, more red cells and hemoglobin, and a high percentage of slow oxidative and fast oxidative glycolytic muscle fibers. Mitochondria, the energy-producing units of muscle and other cells, are inherited from the maternal side. Recent evidence indicates that the capacity of muscle to respond to training is also inherited, with improvements from aerobic training ranging from 5 to over 30 percent (Bouchard

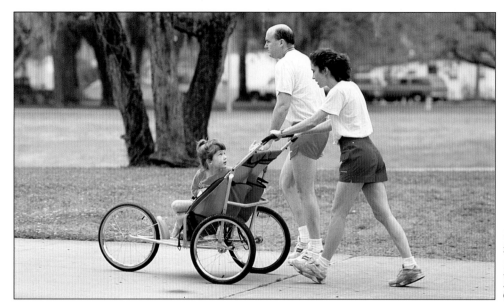

© Anthony Neste

Heredity and environment influence aerobic fitness.

et al. 1988). Other inherited factors such as physique and body composition will also influence the potential to perform at a high level.

Training

The potential to improve aerobic fitness with training is limited; though most studies confirm the potential to improve 20 to 25 percent (more with loss of body fat), only adolescents can hope to improve much more than 30 percent. Consider two individuals, one with an untrained $\dot{V}O_2$max of 40 ml/kg · min, and the other with a score of 60. Let us assume that heredity accounts for the difference in scores. What happens if each trains and gains a 25 percent improvement in $\dot{V}O_2$max?

a. 40 × 25% = 10 + 40 = 50 ml/kg · min

b. 60 × 25% = 15 + 60 = 75 ml/kg · min

Training raises "a" above the average for young men ,whereas "b" is elevated to the level of elite endurance athletes. Even in the untrained state, "b" has a higher $\dot{V}O_2$max than "a" does when trained. Who ever said life was fair?

Training improves the function and capacity of the respiratory and cardiovascular systems and boosts blood volume, but the most important changes take place in the muscle fibers that are used in the training. Aerobic training improves muscles' ability to produce energy aerobically and to metabolize fat. Training makes muscle an efficient furnace for the combustion of fat, producing perhaps the single most important health benefit of regular exercise. Burning fat reduces fat storage, blood fat levels, and cardiovascular risk. It also improves insulin sensitivity and reduces the risk of diabetes. This fat metabolism may also contribute to a lower risk of some cancers. Of course, training enhances the ability to perform, but the improvement is limited to the activity used in training. Long-duration training will increase the aerobic threshold, and higher-intensity effort will raise the lactate threshold. I'll say more about the specificity of training in later chapters.

> Training makes muscle an efficient furnace for the combustion of fat, producing perhaps the single most important health benefit of regular exercise.

5

Aerobic Fitness: The Training Effect

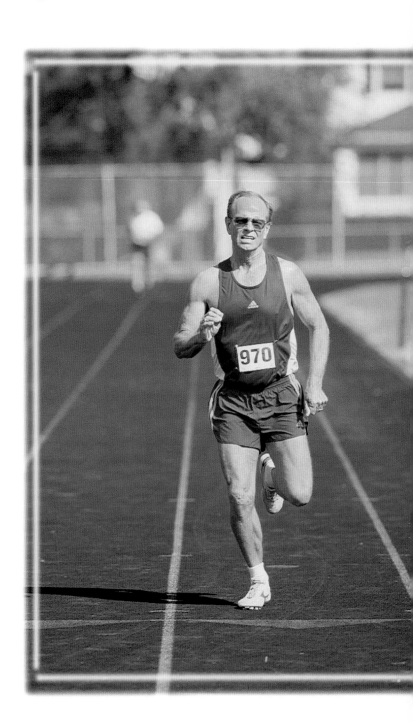

"Nothing in the world can take the place of persistence."

Calvin Coolidge

Years ago, as I began my career in exercise physiology, we used the term *cardiovascular* to define fitness. Next came the term *cardiorespiratory,* and today we speak of *aerobic* fitness. The changes in terminology reflect insights derived from several decades of research, based on a clearer view of the effects of training. We used cardiovascular when the best documented effects of training were on the heart and circulation. Cardiorespiratory became popular when we began to understand the importance of oxygen intake as well as transport. And aerobic was adopted to indicate that oxygen intake, transport, and utilization were all improved with training. Since 1967, when research first documented the effects of endurance training on the muscles' ability to use oxygen, there has been a growing awareness that some of the most important effects of training involve skeletal muscles and their ability to carry out oxidative, or aerobic, energy production. To emphasize that point I like to say that skeletal muscle is the target of training.

You've been told that fitness is good for the heart and the lungs, and that is true. But training requires the use of muscles, and major changes take place in the muscles that are used in training. Of course, important second-ary adaptations take place in the respiratory, cardiovascular, and neuroen-docrine systems and other tissues (fat, bone, ligaments, tendons). But it is impossible to improve the health or function of organs such as the heart without involving the skeletal muscles. All the beneficial changes begin with muscular activity. Train the muscles properly, and the secondary benefits follow; fail to train the muscles, and the other changes are unlikely to occur.

▮ This chapter will help you

- understand how systematic exercise (training) stimulates changes in
  - muscle fibers;
  - respiration and oxygen transport;
  - blood volume;
  - the heart and circulation;
  - the endocrine system;
  - fat metabolism and body composition; and
  - bones, ligaments, and tendons; and
- understand the specificity of training and its importance for the design of effective programs.

The Training Effect

When you engage in an exercise such as walking or jogging at a level above your normal daily activity (load), you *overload* the muscles and their supply and support systems, including the heart and lungs. Repeat the exercise regularly (e.g., every other day) and your body begins to adapt to the overload imposed by the exercise. We call the many adaptations the *training effect.* The exercise some-how signals muscle fibers to undergo changes that will permit more exercise in the future.

The Training Stimulus

Figure 5.1 illustrates the basic structure of a muscle fiber. Something associated with training (metabolic by-products, chemical messenger, hormone) tells the *deoxyribonucleic acid* (DNA) in the muscle fiber's nuclei to produce specific messengers in the form of *ribonucleic acid* (RNA). The messenger RNA (mRNA) travels to structures within the fiber called ribosomes to direct the synthesis of specific proteins, like aerobic enzymes. Transfer RNA (tRNA) reads the mRNA blueprint and then captures appropriate amino acids for use in the synthesis of the desired protein. Endurance training leads to an increase in the concentration of oxidative enzymes and to a rise in the size and number of mitochondria, the cellular power plants where all oxidative metabolism takes place (Hood et al. 2000). These particular adaptations are specific to endurance training, and they take place only in the muscles used in training.

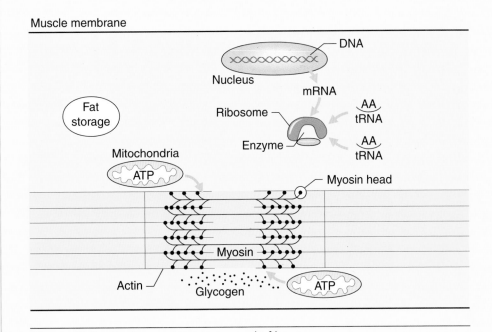

Figure 5.1 Basic structures in a muscle fiber.

In this analysis of the effects of training, I try to rely on studies conducted on humans. A typical study involves pretesting of volunteer subjects for aerobic fitness, lactate threshold, and other measures; random assignment to experimental or control groups; weeks or even months of systematic and progressive training; and posttesting to measure the adaptations due to training. Studies have ranged from low to high intensity, using low- to high-fit subjects. I'll review the effects of aerobic training, then differentiate specific effects of long-slow versus high-intensity training.

A variation of the training study involves *detraining* already-fit subjects. Researchers convince habitual exercisers to forgo training for a period while they observe the decline of important measures and performance. Although this approach has limits, it eliminates the need for prolonged training. We'll look at both types of studies as well as animal research to help you understand the training effect.

Muscle: The Target of Training

The effects of aerobic training on muscle relate to the utilization of oxygen.

Muscle, the motive force and source of many of the good things associated with exercise, is the primary target of training. The effects of aerobic training on muscle relate to the utilization of oxygen. Oxidative metabolism, the enzymatic breakdown of carbohydrate and fat to produce energy for muscular contractions, takes place in cellular powerhouses called mitochondria (Coggan and Williams 1995). Aerobic training has the following effects on muscle:

- It increases the concentration of aerobic enzymes (protein compounds that catalyze metabolic reactions) needed for the metabolic breakdown of carbohydrate and fat to produce energy in the form of ATP (adenosine triphosphate, the cellular energy supply).
- It increases the size and number (volume) of mitochondria, the cellular powerhouses that produce energy aerobically (with oxygen).
- It increases the muscle's ability to use fat as a source of energy.
- It increases the size of the fibers used in training: long-slow training improves the oxidative capabilities of slow oxidative fibers, whereas high-intensity training enhances the capabilities of fast oxidative glycolytic fibers.
- It increases the myoglobin (a compound that carries oxygen from the cell membrane to the mitochondria) content in muscle fibers.
- It increases the number of capillaries serving muscle fibers.

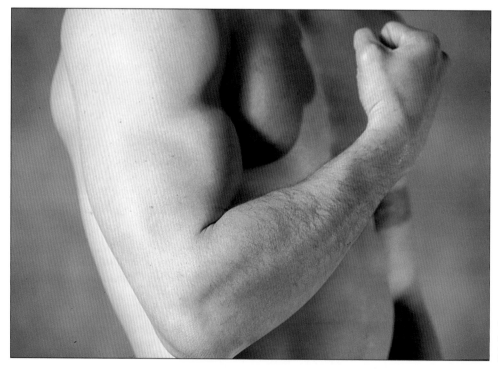

© Action Images

Skeletal muscle is the target of training.

Cellular Effects

Before 1967, research had failed to demonstrate the effects of training on muscle fibers. Dr. John Holloszy reasoned that previous studies failed to overload aerobic pathways, so he subjected laboratory rats to a strenuous treadmill program. Trained rats eventually were able to continue exercise for four to eight hours, whereas untrained animals were exhausted within 30 minutes. Following the 12-week program, the animals were sacrificed to allow study of the muscle tissue. Holloszy found a 50 to 60 percent increase in mitochondrial protein, a twofold rise in the oxygen consumption of trained muscle, and enhanced ability to use (oxidize) carbohydrate and fat (1967). These findings have been replicated in other labs and confirmed in humans, using a muscle biopsy technique. Today we know that the increase in mitochondrial mass is due to branching of existing mitochondria, and that the increase provides greater capacity for oxidation of energy sources, especially our abundant supply of fat (we store 50 times more fat energy than carbohydrate, and training makes that supply more available).

Training Supply and Support Systems

The respiratory, circulatory, nervous, endocrine, and other systems supply and support the activities of muscles. How are they affected by aerobic training? Aerobic training

- increases the efficiency of respiration and the endurance of respiratory muscles;
- improves blood volume, distribution, and delivery to muscles;
- improves cardiovascular efficiency (increases stroke volume and cardiac output while decreasing the resting and exercise heart rates); and
- fine-tunes nervous and hormonal control mechanisms.

Respiration and Oxygen Transport

Aerobic training doesn't alter the size of the lungs, but it does improve the endurance and efficiency of breathing muscles, allowing greater use of inherited capacity (see figure 5.2). Training reduces the residual volume, the portion of lung capacity that goes unused. Residual volume increases with age and inactivity, and this decline of lung volume eventually reduces exercise capacity. The human respiratory system is overbuilt for its task, however, so the gradual decline isn't noticed at first. Aerobic training slows the decline, insuring adequate respiratory capacity throughout life.

Training also enhances the efficiency of respiration, so fewer breaths are needed to move the same volume of air. Ventilation is the amount of air moving in or out of the lungs. It is the product of respiratory rate (or frequency) times the volume of air in each breath (tidal volume).

Ventilation (expired air in liters per minute [L/min])
= Frequency × Tidal volume

Consider values for trained and untrained subjects:

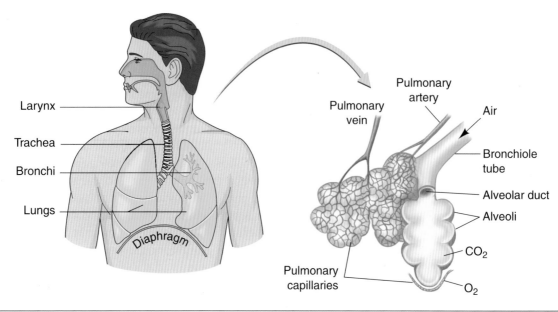

Figure 5.2 Respiratory system.

| Untrained | 60 L/min = 30 breaths × 2 L/breath |
| Trained | 60 L/min = 20 breaths × 3 L/breath |

The trained individual moves more air with fewer breaths and is also able to move more air at maximal ventilation (150 L/min or more, versus 120 or less for the untrained). Slower, deeper breaths are more efficient because they allow more of each breath to reach the portion of the lungs where oxygen and carbon dioxide are exchanged (alveolar sacs). And training improves diffusion of oxygen from the lungs into the blood. Diffusion depends on good ventilation and adequate blood flow in the capillaries.

Blood Volume

It is likely that training-induced changes in blood volume are responsible, at least in part, for so-called cardiovascular changes.

Oxygen is transported via red blood cells and hemoglobin. We have long known that aerobic fitness is closely associated with total hemoglobin, and that blood volume and hemoglobin improve with training. More recently we have learned that the loss of blood volume that occurs with detraining is closely correlated with the reversal of important cardiovascular adjustments (lower heart rate and increased stroke volume) (Coyle, Hemmert, and Coggan 1986). Thus it is likely that training-induced changes in blood volume are responsible, at least in part, for so-called cardiovascular changes, and that these changes may be secondary to changes in blood volume. Blood volume may increase 10 to 15 percent with training, raising the volume from 5 liters to 5.5 or even 5.75 liters. A large portion of the enhanced cardiovascular function of endurance athletes is due to their high blood volume and its effect on cardiac function (Gledhill, Warburton, and Jamnik 1999).

Heart and Circulation

For years we knew that endurance training led to a reduction in the heart rate at rest and at submaximal workloads and to an increase in the stroke volume, the amount of blood pumped with each beat of the heart. That is why we used the term cardiovascular to describe training effects. Training leads to an increase in the size of the left ventricle, but only during the filling stage, or diastole (increased left ventricular end diastolic volume [LVEDV]) (see figure 5.3). This change takes place with some thickening of the heart muscle and subtle alterations in its oxidative enzyme capacity. The efficient trained heart pumps more blood each time it beats, at rest or during exercise, and therefore it can beat at a slower rate. The heart is a pump that ejects much of the blood that enters its chambers; put more blood into the chamber, and more comes out.

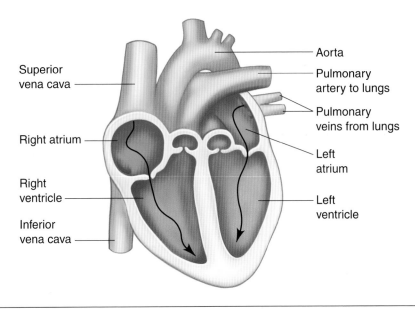

Figure 5.3 The heart.

Stroke Volume

Stroke volume depends on the blood volume and the size of the left ventricle. But the heart is enclosed in a fibrous sac (pericardium) that may limit its size. When the sac was removed from dog hearts, the animals were able to train and increase their stroke volume and cardiac output (cardiac output equals heart rate multiplied by stroke volume) a whopping 20 percent (Stray-Gunderson 1986). You can't risk removal of your pericardium (an infection could lead to heart failure), but you can increase blood volume with training, and that seems to lead to increases in stroke volume and cardiac output and decreases in resting and exercise heart rates. Does the heart rate go down because the stroke volume goes up, or vice versa? You'll soon see.

It appears that aerobic training has subtle effects on the thickness of heart muscle and on aerobic enzymes and mitochondria. The trained heart is better able to use fat as a source of energy, perhaps because training enlarges the diameter of coronary arteries and improves the oxygen supply to heart muscle.

Another important contributor to stroke volume and cardiac output is a redistribution of blood from digestive and other organs to working muscles.

Blood vessels in active muscles dilate whereas those in other organs constrict, directing blood where it is needed during exercise and helping to maintain a high stroke volume. Training actually improves this ability to redistribute blood.

Training also seems to enhance delivery of blood to muscle fibers via the capillaries. Trained muscles have a higher capillary-fiber ratio (Blomqvist and Saltin 1983). Because trained muscle fibers increase in diameter, the rise in capillaries may be necessary to maintain a short diffusion distance from the capillary to the interior of the fiber.

Nervous System

Training has several subtle but important effects on the nervous system. These include improved economy and efficiency of movement and improved efficiency of the cardiovascular system.

The economical athlete uses less energy to perform at a given speed. Hours of practice lead to a relaxed and efficient use of force to achieve results. This economy is especially evident in skilled tasks such as swimming and cross-country skiing, but it can also be found in running or cycling. Trained distance runners use 10 percent less energy than nontrained distance runners to run at a given speed.

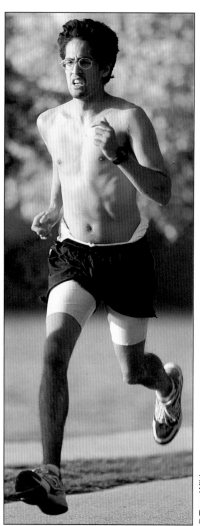

© Terry Wild

The efficient athlete uses less energy to perform at a given speed.

The nervous system, which controls the heart rate and the constriction and relaxation of blood vessels, participates in another adjustment that may help solve the question of why heart rate and stroke volume change with training. In 1977 Saltin published a simple but elegant experiment in which subjects trained one leg on a bicycle ergometer, with the other leg serving as a control (see figure 5.4). Pre- and posttest measures of oxygen intake and oxidative enzyme activity demonstrated that changes occurred only in the trained leg; in other words, that the training was specific. Furthermore, the heart rate response to exercise was significantly lower for the trained leg, but not for the control, or untrained, leg.

Saltin reasoned that the improvements in the trained muscle were responsible for the lower heart rate response. Mitchell and associates (1977) demonstrated that small nerve endings located in muscle fibers are able to sense conditions in the muscle and modify the heart rate response to exercise via connections to the cardiac control center in the brain. Thus it appears that training's influence on the muscle may alter cardiovascular responses—that the reduced heart rate can be traced to the improved metabolic condition in trained muscle. When the heart beats more slowly it has more time to fill, allowing an improved stroke volume.

This interpretation suggests that some of the well-documented effects of training are actually by-products of changes in the skeletal muscles. When we consider these changes with the increase in blood volume and redistribution of blood, which combine to put more blood into the heart, we understand why training leads to a decrease in the exercise heart rate and an increase in the stroke volume. It therefore appears that some so-called cardiovascular effects of training are actually due to changes in the muscles being trained, that these changes are specific, and that training doesn't easily transfer from one leg (or one activity) to another.

Endocrine System

The endocrine system includes the many glands whose secretions—hormones—are distributed via the circulation. The effects of training include

- adjustments in hormonal response,
- increased sensitivity to certain hormones, and
- important metabolic adjustments.

Many hormones are involved in the regulation of energy; epinephrine, cortisol, thyroxine, glucagon, and growth hormone raise blood sugar, whereas insulin is the only hormone capable of lowering blood sugar. Insulin is secreted from the pancreas when blood sugar levels are elevated, such as after a meal, helping tissues take up the sugar. The others are secreted when levels are low, as in vigorous exercise. Epineph-

rine and growth hormone also are involved in the mobilization of fat from adipose tissue, whereas insulin leads to fat deposition. Endurance training lowers the need for insulin because the muscle can take up sugar during exercise, even in the absence of insulin (as in diabetes). Training seems to increase receptor sensitivity to insulin, leading to a more efficient use of hormones and energy.

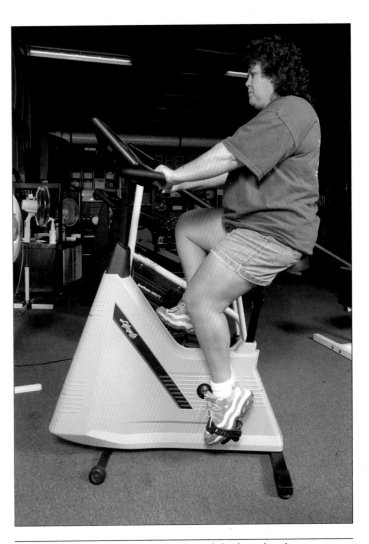

Fat Metabolism

Years ago, animal and then human studies demonstrated improved fat utilization following training. The trained muscle is better suited to use fat as a source of energy, thereby conserving limited supplies of carbohydrate (glycogen) in muscle and the liver. A key finding was the enhancement of beta oxidation, an enzymatic

Figure 5.4 Subject trains one leg while the other leg serves as an untrained control.

process that systematically chops two carbon fragments from fat (free fatty acids). Along with this improvement in fat metabolism is a near doubling of stored fat (triglyceride) in trained muscle fibers. On top of all this, training leads to improvements in fat mobilization.

Fat Mobilization

Epinephrine is available from two sites, the adrenal gland and the nerve endings of the sympathetic nervous system. Like most other hormones, epinephrine acts on receptors located in the surface membrane of its target organ, in this case adipose tissue. The hormone initiates a series of steps leading to the breakdown of triglyceride fat and the release of free fatty acids (FFA) into the circulation (see figure 5.5). The FFA then travel to working muscles or the heart, where they can be used to fuel contractions. During very vigorous exercise, lactic acid produced in the muscles seems to inhibit the action of epinephrine, thereby reducing the FFA available for energy. Under these conditions the muscle is forced to use limited supplies of muscle glycogen for energy.

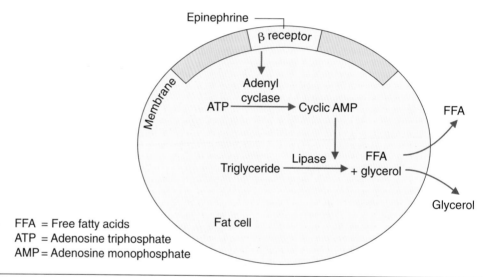

Figure 5.5 Mobilization of free fatty acids from adipose tissue. Lactic acid inhibits the influence of epinephrine on the fat cell and blocks the mobilization of fat.

Adapted from Sharkey 1990.

I'll say it again: The ability to utilize fat may be one of the most important outcomes of the active life and fitness.

Training improves the oxidative ability of muscles, leading to less lactic acid production and greater fat mobilization and fat metabolism (Holloszy et al. 1986). And it appears that trained individuals are able to mobilize fat even when lactic acid is elevated (Vega deJesus and Siconolfi 1988). The result is improved access to a major source of energy, some 50 times more abundant than carbohydrate! And the enhanced utilization of fat has significant health benefits as well as those related to fitness and performance. I'll say it again: The ability to utilize fat may be one of the most important outcomes of the active life and fitness.

Other Effects of Training

Training has effects on other tissues, including adipose tissue (fat), bone, ligaments, and tendons. Though some are mere adjustments that counteract the stresses of training, making more activity possible, others have health and cosmetic effects.

Body Composition

Body composition refers to the relative amounts of fat and lean weight. Although the lean body weight (body weight minus fat weight) is relatively unchanged with aerobic training, substantial loss of fat tissue is to be expected. One of the best documented effects of training is the loss of unwanted fat and a change in body composition, revealing a trim, pleasing figure. Researchers use underwater weighing or skinfold calipers to measure percent body fat.

If you have 25 percent fat and weigh 120 pounds (54.4 kilograms), you have 30 pounds (13.6 kilograms) of fat and 90 pounds (40.8 kilograms) of lean body weight (LBW). If you jog 3 miles (4.8 kilometers) a day, five days a week, you will burn about 1,650 calories per week (3 miles times 110 calories per mile times five days equals 1,650 calories). In just two weeks you'll burn 3,300 extra calories, almost a pound of fat (3,500 calories equals one pound [.45 kilograms] of fat), or almost two pounds (.9 kilograms) a month. In the process you will lower your percent body fat and your body weight with only a slight increase in LBW. I'll say more about body composition and fat loss in chapters 12 and 13.

Bones, Ligaments, and Tendons

Bones, ligaments, and tendons respond to the stresses placed on them. Every change in function is followed by adaptations. For bones, increased activity leads to a denser, stronger structure designed to counteract the new level of stress. Inactivity leads to reabsorption of calcium and loss of supportive structures. Increasing age and inactivity create a dangerous combination, especially for females. Bone demineralization, or osteoporosis, begins early in adult life (30 to 40 years of age) and becomes more serious after menopause. Lack of activity hastens the weakening of bones. And though moderate activity causes bone tissue to become stronger and more dense, excessive training associated with weight loss or menstrual irregularities (amenorrhea, or absence of menstruation) can cause early and possibly irreversible osteoporosis. Calcium intake may be helpful, but it won't do much good without the stress of moderate weight-bearing exercise.

Moderate activity also strengthens ligaments, tendons, and other connective tissue, such as the covering of muscle. By gradually increasing the workload, you can make tissues tough enough to withstand the normal demands of activity and to resist damage during slips, trips, and falls.

Specificity of Training

The outcomes of training are directly related to the activity employed as a training stimulus.

An activity such as jogging recruits muscle fibers uniquely suited to the task. Slow fibers are recruited for slow jogging. The metabolic pathways and energy sources are also suited to the task. Daily jogging recruits the same fibers and pathways over and over, leading to the adaptive response known as the training effect.

The outcomes of training are directly related to the activity employed as a training stimulus. We've shown that training has effects on muscle fibers as well as on the supply and support systems, such as the respiratory and cardiovascular systems. In general, the effects of training on muscle fibers are very specific, meaning that they are unlikely to transfer to activities unlike the training. So most of the benefits of run training will not transfer to swimming or cycling. On the other hand, the effects on the respiratory or cardiovascular systems are more general, so they may transfer to other activities (Sharkey and Greatzer 1993).

Training leads to changes in aerobic enzyme systems in muscle fibers, so it is easy to see why those changes are specific. In the early stages of training, the muscles' inability to use oxygen limits performance. Later on, as the fibers adapt and can utilize more oxygen, the burden shifts to the cardiovascular system, including the heart, blood, and blood vessels. Then the cardiovascular system becomes the factor that limits performance (Boileau, McKeown, and Riner 1984).

Training gains don't automatically transfer from one activity to another. Training effects can be classified as *peripheral* (in the muscle) and *central* (heart, blood, lungs, hormones). Central effects may transfer to other activities, but peripheral changes are unlikely to transfer. However, central changes in blood volume and redistribution may aid performance in another endurance activity. But keep in mind that one-leg training studies show that some part of the heart rate (and stroke volume) change is due to conditions within the muscle fibers, conditions that are relayed to the cardiac control center (Saltin 1977). These changes are specific and will not transfer from one activity to another.

It makes sense to concentrate training on the movements, muscle fibers, metabolic pathways, and supply and support systems that you intend to use in the activity or sport. This does not imply that athletes should ignore other exercises and muscle groups. Additional training is necessary to avoid injury, to avoid boredom, to achieve muscle balance, and to provide backup for prime movers when they become fatigued. In spite of the widespread affection for the term cardiovascular fitness, the evidence suggests that the concept is overrated. Muscle is the target of training.

Finally, if exercise and training are specific, it stands to reason that testing must be specific if it is to reflect the adaptations to training. This means you should not use a bicycle to test a runner, and vice versa. Training is so specific that hill runners are best tested on an uphill treadmill test. How do we test the effects of training on dancers? We don't. When studies compare runners and dancers on a treadmill test, the runners exhibit higher $\dot{V}O_2$max scores. If that is true, why do runners poop out in aerobic dance, cycling, or swimming? Because the effects of training are specific. At present there is no widely accepted way to accurately assess the effects of aerobic, ballet, modern, or other dance forms.

Summary

In this section we've looked at the effects of aerobic training. I've shown that muscles undergo specific adaptations when they are recruited in exercise that lasts long enough to overload their oxidative pathways. As aerobic pathways are improved, muscles use oxygen more efficiently and burn more fat, and the lactate threshold is raised. The metabolic efficiency is relayed to the cardiac control center in the brain, which results in a slower heart rate, more filling time, and a greater stroke volume. Increased blood volume and improved distribution provide ample blood for the heart to pump. Because so many adaptations take place in the muscle, training should be specific to its intended use.

Because training is so specific, it is important that you select an appropriate activity for aerobic training. Fat metabolism and cardiovascular benefits are enhanced in regular moderate activity that employs major muscle groups for extended periods, but not when different muscles are engaged in a series of short lifting bouts (i.e., circuit weight training). Bone mineral content is maintained when bones are subjected to regular moderate stress, as in weight-bearing and resistance exercises.

Choose an activity you enjoy, or one you want to improve. Long-slow training improves the ability of slow oxidative fibers to use fat as an energy source. Faster and necessarily shorter training recruits fast-twitch (fast oxidative glycolytic) fibers. High-intensity training may also have more effect on the cardiovascular system. Your approach to training depends on your goals. Train more slowly for distance, faster for speed. You can combine both by going easy and then increasing pace near the end of the workout. German distance coach Ernst Van Aaken advocated a 20:1 slow:fast ratio for his elite athletes (1976). For example, on a 5-mile (8-kilometer) run, pick up the pace for the last quarter-mile (the last 0.4 kilometer). This short distance provides some speed training at a time when you are well warmed. I like this approach because it limits the discomfort associated with elevated lactic acid. Training doesn't have to hurt to be good.

6

Improving Aerobic Fitness

"Fitness can neither be bought nor bestowed. Like honor it must be earned."

Anonymous

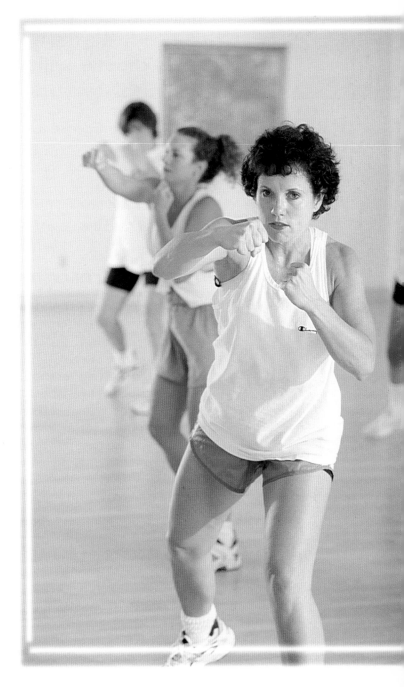

Years ago, before we knew how to prescribe exercise, we were faced with a number of unproven training systems that were based on the ideas and experience of well-known physicians, coaches, or educators. Then researchers began to identify the factors associated with improvements in fitness. Today's exercise prescriptions are based on the results of hundreds of studies. The dose of exercise that safely promotes the training effect is usually represented in terms of the intensity, duration, and frequency of exercise. Research and clinical experience are adding to a carefully developed methodology for the safe and effective prescription of exercise.

Aerobic fitness is earned minute by minute, day by day, as you engage in appropriate training exercises. As with any treatment or drug, the exercises must be prescribed and taken with care if the benefits are to be realized and if potentially harmful side effects are to be avoided.

▌ This chapter will help you

- utilize your heart rate or perceived exertion to determine exercise intensity;
- determine exercise duration using calories, minutes, or miles (kilometers);
- decide on the appropriate frequency of exercise;
- develop a personalized aerobic fitness prescription based on your level of fitness and training goals; and
- understand how to achieve, maintain, and regain aerobic fitness.

The Fitness Prescription

Throughout history people have sought the health benefits believed to be associated with exercise, with prescriptions dating back to centuries-old Chinese and Roman documents. In the late 1800s Dr. Dudley Sargent, physician and director of the Harvard College Gymnasium, tested students and prescribed exercises to rectify weaknesses. Prescriptions improved only slightly until the 1950s, when researchers began to establish the link between lack of activity and heart disease. Since then, we have agreed on a definition of aerobic fitness, identified the factors that contribute to its improvement, and become more aware of the benefits and limitations of exercise as a modality for disease prevention and rehabilitation. We now know how hard (intensity), how long (duration), and how often (frequency) one must exercise to achieve an aerobic training effect. We'll discuss the prescription, then learn how to proceed.

Intensity

Intensity is the most important factor in the development of maximal oxygen intake ($\dot{V}O_2max$); it reflects the energy requirements of the exercise, the amount of oxygen consumed, and the calories of energy expended. Though intensity is usually defined with the training heart rate, other measures can also be used (see table 6.1).

Table 6.1 Measures of Exercise Intensity[a]

Intensity	Heart rate (bpm)	$\dot{V}O_2$ (L/min)	Cal/min[b]	METs[c]
Light	100	1.0	5	4.0
Moderate	135	2.0	10	8.1
Heavy	170	3.0	15	12.2

The number of calories burned per minute depends on body weight; therefore, a heavier individual burns more during a given exercise. Each MET equals 3.5 ml/kg · min, so the MET is adjusted for body weight. The aerobics point system popularized by Dr. Kenneth Cooper is a close relative of the MET. Each aerobic point is worth 7 ml/kg · min, or 2 METs.

[a]For 70-kg individual, fitness score = 45.

[b]1 L of oxygen is equivalent to 5 cal/min.

[c]The MET, or metabolic equivalent, is a multiple of the resting metabolic rate. The resting rate is 1.2 cal/min (1 MET), so 12 cal/min = 10 METs.

Training Heart Rate

Early training studies focused on the metabolic demands of training (liters of oxygen or kilocalories of energy expenditure). The heart rate was used as a simple, inexpensive way to translate training information to the lay public—merely a by-product of the metabolic activity. Unfortunately, over the years the public and some fitness professionals have lost sight of this point. Today many mistakenly consider the training heart rate, and not the sustained metabolism of a large muscle mass (e.g., legs), to be the goal of training. They believe that raising the heart rate, no matter how it is done, will result in improvements in fitness. For example, the elevation of the heart rate during weight training has led some to believe that circuit weight training could be used to improve aerobic fitness. They ignore the fact that each muscle group is engaged for only 20 to 30 seconds, far too short a time to prompt changes in the oxidative pathways of muscles. The training heart rate is a convenient external indicator of exercise intensity and oxygen consumption, but it isn't an end in itself. I'll say more about the real target of training later in this chapter.

Aerobic Threshold

Early training studies agreed that training had to exceed a certain minimum level or threshold if significant changes in fitness were to occur (see figure 6.1).

In one study we trained young men at heart rates of 120, 150, and 180 beats per minute (bpm). The higher-intensity groups improved similarly, but the low-intensity subjects did not (Sharkey and Holleman 1967). Then we learned that training intensity depended on one's level of fitness, with low-fit subjects making progress at lower intensities while high-fit subjects had a higher training threshold (Sharkey 1970). The minimal training threshold is called the aerobic threshold.

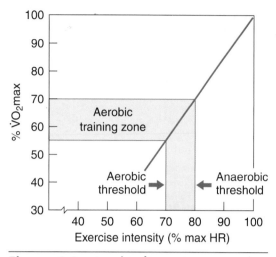

Figure 6.1 Aerobic fitness improves when you exercise within the aerobic training zone.

Anaerobic (Lactate) Threshold

Studies also defined an upper limit to training intensity. They showed that training above that level didn't yield additional benefits. In recent years we recognized that the upper limit of the training zone coincides with the anaerobic, or lactate, threshold. When the activity exceeds the muscle's ability to produce energy aerobically and blood lactate begins to accumulate, the exercise's contribution to aerobic fitness diminishes. Stated another way, anaerobic exercise does not contribute substantially to the development of aerobic fitness.

Thus there is an aerobic training zone that ranges from the aerobic threshold on the low end to the anaerobic (lactate) threshold, the point of diminishing returns. Training at the low end of the zone leads to improvements in fat metabolism and changes in slow oxidative muscle fibers. Training at the high end of the zone recruits and benefits fast oxidative glycolytic muscle fibers and leads to central circulatory (cardiovascular) benefits. Also, the high-intensity interval training athletes use has been shown to raise the anaerobic (lactate) threshold. This improvement sometimes takes place without an increase in the $\dot{V}O_2$max, especially in athletes who have already undergone extensive training.

> Stated another way, anaerobic exercise does not contribute substantially to the development of aerobic fitness.

The Training Zone

Both thresholds are related to your level of activity and fitness. Inactive individuals have a low aerobic threshold. If normal daily activity seldom exceeds a slow walk, a brisk walk will exceed the threshold and elicit a training effect. Regular participation in high-intensity activity raises the anaerobic threshold, so highly active individuals have an elevated threshold and a higher training zone.

The training zone is based on a percentage of your estimated maximal heart rate (max HR). Because the max HR declines with age, we use both fitness level and the age-adjusted max HR to determine the training zone.

Fitness (ml/kg · min)	Training zone (% max HR)
Low (under 35)	60 to 75 percent
Medium (35 to 45)	70 to 85 percent
High (over 45)	75 to 90 percent

If your max HR hasn't been measured, estimate it with the formula: max HR equals 220 minus age. Because there is considerable variability in the estimation of the max HR (see chapter 3), you should view the estimated HR with caution. If your training zone feels too high, back off to a more comfortable level. Your max HR may be lower than expected. If it feels far too easy, move it up a bit. Because of this variability I like to use the rating of perceived exertion (RPE) along with the training zone.

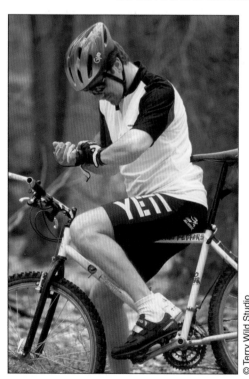

© Terry Wild Studio

Use your heart rate as a measure of exercise intensity.

Table 6.2 Borg's RPE Scale

6	No exertion at all
7	Extremely light
8	
9	Very light
10	
11	Light
12	
13	Somewhat hard
14	
15	Hard (heavy)
16	
17	Very hard
18	
19	Extremely hard
20	Maximal exertion

Borg RPE scale
© Gunnar Borg, 1970, 1985, 1994, 1998

The RPE is a simple 20-point rating scale designed to provide an estimate of exercise intensity (see table 6.2).

The data from a large multicenter research project indicate that the RPE can also be used to estimate the aerobic and anaerobic (lactate) thresholds (Gaskill et al. 2001).

Aerobic threshhold	RPE = 11	Light
Anaerobic threshold	RPE = 15/16	Hard

The numbers in the Borg scale are also related to the exercise heart rate; a 15 on the scale approximates a heart rate of 150 (just add a zero to the rating). The "talk test" is another way to determine if you are within your zone. You should be able to carry on a conversation while you train, at least until you approach your lactate threshold. Exercise doesn't have to hurt to be good.

Heart Rate Range

A percentage of your max HR (e.g., 70 percent) is not equivalent to the same percentage of your maximal oxygen intake ($\dot{V}O_2$max). The heart rate range formula calculates a heart rate that is equal to the same percentage of the $\dot{V}O_2$max. For a heart rate that is equivalent to 70 percent of the $\dot{V}O_2$max:

HR = [70% × (max HR – resting HR)] + resting HR

= [70% × (170 – 70)] + 70

= 140 bpm

By contrast, 70 percent of the max HR (170) equals 119 bpm, which is approximately equal to 55 percent of the $\dot{V}O_2$max. The heart rate range is sometimes used to adjust for measured differences in the resting and maximal heart rates, and to avoid errors in the estimation of the training heart rate.

In time you won't need to check your heart rate because you'll know how it feels to be in the training zone (perceived exertion). We begin with a prescription, but as you learn more about exercise and your body, improve your fitness, and decide on your goals, you will outgrow the need for heart rates and training zones. The RPE is a simple way to judge exercise intensity on a numerical scale that is correlated to heart rate and other physiological variables. It has been shown to be a valid tool for the prescription of exercise (Steed, Gaesser, and Weltman 1994).

Duration

Exercise duration and intensity go hand in hand; an increase in one requires a decrease in the other. *Duration* can be prescribed in terms of time, distance, or calories. I mention all three to show how they relate, but I prefer to use the calorie because it is so educational. Food labels tell you how many calories you gain when you eat and drink (double burger equals 550, beer equals 150 calories). You should also know how much exercise it takes to balance your energy intake (over 100 calories per mile [1.6 kilometers] of jogging, so you'd have to jog almost 7 miles [11.2 kilometers] to burn the calories consumed with the beer and burger). It makes you think!

The Calorie

The calorie (technically a kilocalorie) is a unit of energy defined as the amount of heat required to raise the temperature of one kilogram of water one degree Celsius. We store calories when we eat and burn them when we exercise. Caloric expenditure during exercise is influenced by body weight. A 180-pound (81.6-kilogram) person burns more calories running at a certain pace than one who weighs 150 pounds, or 68 kilograms (136 calories per mile [per 1.6 kilometers] versus 113 calories per mile for a 150-pound person). In this book caloric expenditures are based on a weight of 150 pounds; add or subtract 10 percent for each 15 pounds (6.8 kilograms) over or under 150 pounds. For example, add 20 percent to 113 calories to determine the cost for the 180-pound example (113 times .20 equals 22.6, plus 113 equals 135.6 calories).

An early training study showed that low-fit individuals can improve their fitness with as little as 100 calories of exercise per session (10 minutes at 10 calories per minute) (Bouchard et al. 1966). Low-fit subjects do not respond to long-duration or high-intensity training. But in time, as fitness improves, they should extend duration to 200 calories or more. Fitness pioneer Dr. Tom Cureton found that higher expenditures were needed to bring about significant changes in cholesterol levels (Cureton 1969). And more recent studies have shown that longer workouts (more than 35 minutes) produce greater fitness benefits (Wenger and Bell 1986), perhaps because the proportion of fat metabolized continues to rise for the first 30 minutes of exercise.

A study of 17,000 Harvard graduates provides another way to assess the importance of exercise duration. Paffenbarger, Hyde, and Wing (1986) found a significant reduction in the risk of heart disease for graduates who averaged more than 2,000 calories of exercise per week. That translates into about 300 calories daily (400 calories per day in 5 days of exercise, etc.). Longer-duration training leads to improved fat metabolism, which may be the major health benefit of exercise. Increase duration to gain significant fitness, weight control, and fat metabolism benefits and to lower blood lipids. However, there is no conclusive evidence to recommend workouts that exceed 60 minutes (or 600 calories). Endurance athletes participate in longer workouts to improve stamina and performance, not for enhanced health benefits. In fact, a recent study suggests that mortality rates, which decline with exercise, start to rise when energy expenditure rises above 3,500 calories per week (Lee, Hsieh, and Paffenbarger 1995).

Fitness (ml/kg · min)	Duration (cal/session)
Low (under 35)	100 to 200
Medium (35 to 45)	200 to 400
High (over 45)	Over 400

Overload is the key to improvements in training. As fitness improves we need to increase intensity and duration if we hope to continue improvements in $\dot{V}O_2$max and the lactate threshold. Now let's see how training frequency must be adjusted as training progresses.

Frequency

For low-fit individuals, three sessions a week on alternating days are sufficient to improve aerobic fitness (Jackson, Sharkey, and Johnston 1968). But as training progresses in intensity and duration, it must also increase in frequency if improvements are to continue (Pollock 1973). An extensive review of training studies found that changes in fitness are directly related to frequency of training when it is considered independent of the effects of intensity, duration, program length, and initial level of fitness (Wenger and Bell 1986). Six days per week is more than twice as effective as three. So for fitness or weight control, consider more frequent exercise. Athletes engage in long sessions, or they train two or more times a day, two or three times a week. But they also observe the hard-easy principle, following hard or long sessions with easy or short ones. Failure to allow adequate time for recovery from training nullifies its effects; overtraining can lead to poor performances, overuse injuries, or illness via suppression of the immune system.

The body needs time to respond to the training stimulus, and some people find they need more than 24 hours. As I reached my 60th year I found that I needed more time to recover from extremely long or strenuous activity. Experiment with schedules to find one that suits you. Work out daily if you prefer, or try an alternate-day plan and increase duration. Whatever you do, be sure to schedule at least one day of relative rest or diversion each week. A colleague and former training partner once wrote, "We should approach running not as if we are trying to smash our way through some enormous wall, but as a gentle pastime by which

Overtraining can lead to poor performances, overuse injuries, or illness via suppression of the immune system.

we can coax a slow continuous stream of adaptations out of the body" (Frederick 1973:20).

Fitness (ml/kg · min)	Frequency (days per week)
Low (under 35)	3 to 4
Medium (35 to 45)	5 to 6
High (over 45)	More than 6*

*Athletes often do two sessions per day.

Now let's put all the factors together in your personalized prescription for fitness.

Your Prescription

A comprehensive review of training studies showed that maximal gains in aerobic fitness ($\dot{V}O_2$max) were achieved with high intensity (90 percent of $\dot{V}O_2$max or 95 percent of max HR), a duration of 35 to 45 minutes, and a frequency of four times per week (Wenger and Bell 1986). Lesser intensities produced very respectable results with less risk of injury. But keep in mind that all these conclusions were based on changes in the $\dot{V}O_2$max, acknowledged as a measure of intensity (Sharkey 1991). Although $\dot{V}O_2$max is important, there are even better measures of endurance, such as the aerobic or the anaerobic (lactate) thresholds. And fitness and performance aren't the only goals; health benefits, weight control, and improved appearance may be achieved with lower levels of intensity, duration, and frequency. Use the prescription in table 6.3 as a starting point, but don't be a slave to training. Adapt the program to meet your personal style and goals.

Athletes will occasionally train at higher intensities and longer durations and will sometimes do two or even three workouts a day. Chapter 16 provides advice on advanced endurance training and insights into cross-training and other ways to make fitness enjoyable. Table 6.4 shows how some popular training activities fit the prescription.

Figure 6.2 illustrates how the prescription is carried out on a given day. Begin every session with a warm-up to minimize soreness and the risk of injury. Start with a gradual increase in exercise activity, and then stretch. Pay attention to stretching the lower back, hamstrings, calf muscles, and any sore muscles. Muscle soreness shows up 24 hours after the start of a program but diminishes soon thereafter. It won't return unless you lay off for weeks or do a new activity. Follow the prescription during the aerobic portion of the session, then be sure to cool down before you hit the shower. Easy jogging, walking, and stretching help lower

Table 6.3 The Aerobic Fitness Prescription

Fitness (ml/kg · min)	Intensity (% max HR)	Duration (calories)	Frequency (days/wk)
Low (under 35)	60-75	100-200	3-4
Medium (35-45)	70-85	200-400	5-6
High (over 45)	75-90	400+	6+

Table 6.4 Sample Aerobic Activities

Fitness category (ml/kg · min)[a]	Running Distance (mi)[b]	Running Time (min)	Jogging Distance (mi)	Jogging Time (min)	Cycling Distance (mi)	Cycling Time (min)	Walking Distance (mi)	Walking Time (min)
Low (under 35)	0.8-1.7	7-14	0.8-1.7	10-20	1.9-3.9	12-24	1.0-2.1	18-36
Medium (35-45)	1.7-3.4	14-27	1.7-3.4	20-40	3.9-7.8	24-47	2.1-4.2	36-72
High (over 45)	3.4+	27+	3.4+	40+	7.8+	47+	4.2+	72+

[a]Distance and time remain the same regardless of age.
[b]1 mile = 1.6 km

Adapted from Sharkey 1997b.

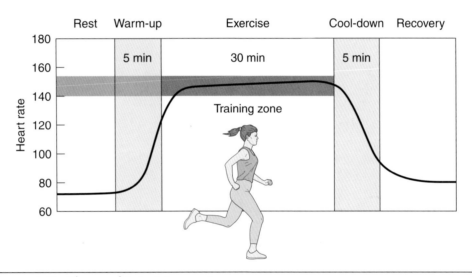

Figure 6.2 The aerobic training session.

the body temperature, reduce metabolic by-products such as lactic acid, and dissipate the hormone norepinephrine, which could cause irregular heart rhythms.

To vary the program, take different routes, work at the upper edge of the zone for shorter periods (i.e., hard-short) and the lower edge for longer periods (easy-long), or use another activity for variety (cross-training). As training progresses, the same pace will feel easier and more enjoyable. As fitness improves, the prescription changes, calling for more intensity, duration, or frequency. By then you will have an idea of what you want to achieve from fitness, and you can decide what works and feels best to you.

In Review

A nomogram developed by Dr. Jeffrey Broida (see figure 6.3) helps you see how intensity, duration, and frequency interact. It shows how you can vary your program to meet your daily and weekly caloric expenditure goals.

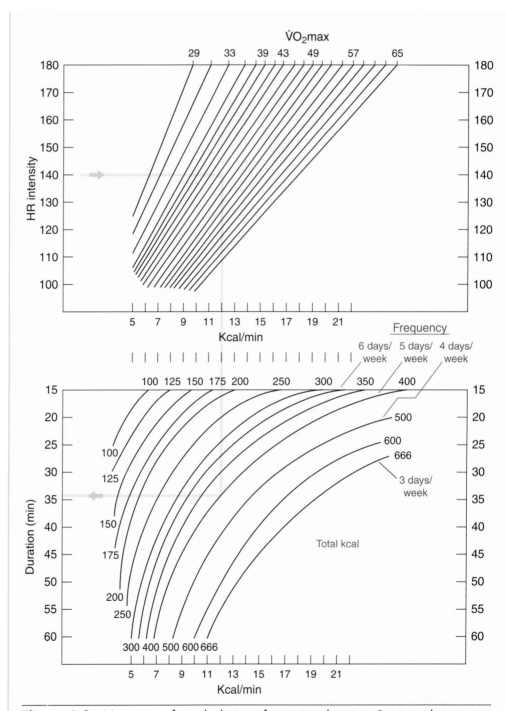

Figure 6.3 Nomogram for calculation of exercise duration. Begin with intensity, move across to fitness level ($\dot{V}O_2$max), then move down to total calories and across to duration (min).

To use the nomogram, choose a heart rate within your training zone and draw a horizontal line connecting with your fitness level. A vertical line indicates your caloric expenditure (calories per minute) at that heart rate. Then drop to the lower graph and intersect the line that describes your daily caloric expenditure goal. Finally, draw a horizontal line to the left until it indicates exercise duration in minutes. In our example in the figure, a 40-year-old with a fitness score of 45 and a training HR of 140 needs 400 calories, which can be achieved with less than 35 minutes of exercise at that intensity. The nomogram also shows several ways to get at least 2,000 calories per week, using more days and shorter sessions or fewer days and longer sessions. Dr. Broida chooses the 2,000-calorie-per-week level for the subject in the example because it has been associated with a lower risk of heart disease. Use the top portion of the nomogram to determine caloric expenditure at a given heart rate and how it increases with training. You burn 12 calories per minute at a heart rate of 140 and a fitness score ($\dot{V}O_2$max) of 47; raise your fitness to 57, and the caloric expenditure is over 15 calories per minute at the same heart rate!

Mode of Exercise

Health benefits occur regardless of the exercise you select. Dr. Michael Pollock and associates compared the fitness and weight-control benefits of walking, running, and cycling. Sedentary middle-aged men trained for 20 weeks, all using the same prescription. Tests administered at the conclusion of the study indicated that all three groups improved similarly in fitness, body weight, and fat (Pollock et al. 1975). No one mode of exercise is superior to others when the prescription is the same. The best exercise is the one you enjoy and will continue to do regularly. However, as discussed earlier, improvements in fitness are specific to the manner of training. So if you want to improve your running, that is the way you should train. Swimming and cycling do surprisingly little to improve running, and vice versa, because many of the really important changes take place only in the muscles used in training.

Cross-Training

The popular triathlon gave rise to the "theory" of cross-training, and the suggestion that running or cycling could enhance swim performance, and so forth. Unfortunately, cross-training doesn't work that way; training must be specific to improve performance (Sharkey and Greatzer 1993). But there are several good reasons to use variety in training. One is to train for a multisport event like the triathlon. Another is to add variety and interest to your training. But the most important reason is to reduce impact and overuse in activities like running.

I run year-round, even in the dead of the Montana winter. I've found that cross-training relieves the likelihood of nagging overuse injuries. And the variety eliminates the boredom of unrelenting training. I run and mountain bike in the summer, with hiking, paddling, swimming, and golf for diversion. The winter includes cross-country and downhill skiing as well as running. Winter diversions include back-country ski trips. I do one or two weightlifting sessions most weeks to maintain muscular fitness and to try to improve or maintain performance. Fall and spring serve as transition periods, enhanced by new activities, new weather, and new locales. Try more than one mode of exercise to train some muscles while resting others. You'll like it!

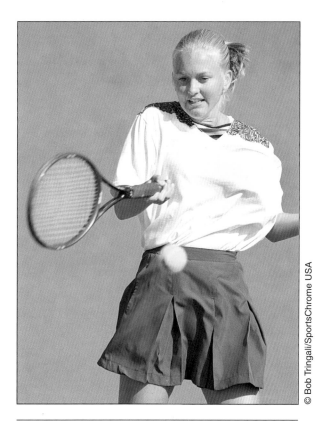

The best exercise is the one you enjoy and continue to do regularly.

It takes time to coax that slow, continuous stream of adaptations from the body.

Achievement

The key to the achievement of fitness goals is to make haste slowly. Rush the process, and the result may be painful, injurious, or worse. It takes time to coax that slow, continuous stream of adaptations from the body. You'll experience improved energy and vigor within weeks, improved self-concept and body image will follow, and performance will show change within a month. But don't view these exciting changes as a license for imprudent behavior. Athletes train for years to achieve dramatic results. Why, then, do older, less-adaptable adults attempt to undo years of inactivity or expect to remove a decade's accumulation of fat in a few short weeks?

What progress can you expect when you follow your prescription? Although the ultimate achievement will depend on your genetic endowment (Bouchard et al. 1988), with time and effort you can achieve your potential. The rate of improvement is influenced by two factors, age and initial level of fitness (Sharkey 1970). Training during or just after puberty, a period of intense growth and development, leads to the greatest adaptations in your ability to take in, transport, and utilize oxygen. Adolescent training may prompt a 30 to 35 percent improvement in aerobic fitness. Young adults are able to improve 20 to 25 percent. Trainability may decline slowly thereafter, but even a 70-year-old can expect a 10 percent improvement in fitness ($\dot{V}O_2$max). Greater improvements are possible at any age when significant weight loss is involved (Sharkey 1984).

Because active individuals are closer to their genetic potential, they will not improve as much as their less-active and less-fit contemporaries. Complete inactivity, such as prolonged bed rest, provides a clean canvas for the demonstration of dramatic changes, perhaps as much as 100 percent improvement above bed rest levels. Sedentary folks may improve over 30 percent, whereas already trained athletes may have to accept 5 percent improvement or less, depending on age, proximity to genetic potential, and level of training.

The rate of improvement is dramatic at first, 3 percent per week for the first month, 2 percent per week for the second, and slowing to 1 percent or less thereafter. But even though the improvements in aerobic fitness begin to plateau after several months, the capacity to perform submaximal work continues to grow (see figure 6.4). Both the capacity for prolonged work (aerobic threshold) and the upper limit of aerobic endurance (lactate threshold) continue to increase after the $\dot{V}O_2$max has plateaued. And it is these submaximal capacities and not the $\dot{V}O_2$max that define our capacity for work or sport.

A normally active middle-aged adult male with a fitness score of 40 ml/kg · min may improve to 50. If he had started as an adolescent, with a fitness score of 55, and achieved a 30 percent improvement, he may have scored over 70 and been an

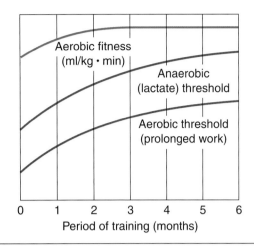

Figure 6.4 Training, aerobic fitness, and submaximal work capacity. With prolonged training, aerobic fitness begins to plateau, but the capacity to perform submaximal work continues to improve.

outstanding athlete. If you started late, don't despair; you can still achieve dramatic improvements in endurance and energy. Most important are the improvements in the submaximal capacities, changes that allow a once-sedentary individual to climb a mountain or run a marathon. In addition to improvements in fitness, you are able to sustain a higher percentage of your max and continue once-fatiguing activities indefinitely, without fatigue or discomfort. And the benefits will extend beyond your regular mode of exercise to all your daily tasks. Fitness expands your horizons.

Maintenance

If you attain a level of fitness and performance that meets your needs, you may want to switch to a maintenance program. You'll be able to maintain your fitness with three sessions per week, allowing time to apply your newfound fitness in new pursuits. Maintenance has been studied several ways. One is to train to a level of fitness, then use various frequencies of training to see how much is required to remain at that level. Another is to cease training to see how quickly fitness is lost. With some activity, fitness doesn't decline too rapidly, but with complete bed rest it may drop as much as 10 percent a week (Greenleaf et al. 1976). You can maintain fitness with two or three sessions weekly, but the effort must be of the same intensity and duration as that used to achieve the improvements (Brynteson and Sinning 1973). Exercise of lower intensity but longer duration also seems to work, but it won't keep you tuned for a race. One workout of very long duration each week may help maintain fitness for a while; a combination of activities plus two or three training sessions is certain to do the job.

More recently, researchers have used a more complex approach to study maintenance. By observing the effect of a single dose of training on specific aerobic enzymes, the researcher can plot the influence of training and determine its half-life, that is, the time it takes to lose one-half of the benefit. These studies suggest that the half-life of training ranges from 4.5 to 9.4 days (Watson, Srivastava, and Booth 1983). The half-life is used because it is difficult to tell when a biological effect, such as an increase in enzyme activity, returns to pretraining levels. So the increase is measured, along with the time it takes to return to half of that value.

If half of the training effect is lost in 4.5 days, you'll want to train more frequently to maintain or improve fitness.

Regaining Fitness

Does a previously fit individual regain fitness more quickly than one who has not been fit? Although the limited work in this area says probably not, my experience argues for a tentative maybe. The answer may depend on such factors as genetic potential, the level of fitness, and the extent of previous training. An extensive period of previous training may lead to changes that are retained longer than alterations in aerobic enzymes and blood volume. And the repetition of training will certainly lead to skill and economy of motion that makes subsequent activity seem easier.

But instead of worrying about how little it takes to achieve, maintain, or regain fitness, find activities you enjoy and make them part of your life. Then you'll view activity as an essential and enjoyable part of every day. You'll be hooked on activity and fitness, and the rest will take care of itself.

Summary

This chapter summarizes the findings of hundreds of studies that have contributed to our knowledge of the factors associated with the development of aerobic fitness. Intensity, duration, and frequency of exercise are manipulated to bring about improvements in fitness. Until recently, virtually all of the studies relied on the same measure of improvement, the $\dot{V}O_2max$, which has been acknowledged as a measure of exercise intensity. So it is not surprising that most studies favor intensity as the most important factor in the training prescription. If your goal is to raise the $\dot{V}O_2max$, by all means emphasize intensity (e.g., the training heart rate), at least some of the time.

However, if your goal is health, or the capacity to endure for extended periods, you should give equal attention to another important dimension of fitness—duration, as measured by the aerobic and lactate (anaerobic) thresholds. Long-duration exercise raises the aerobic threshold and ensures the utilization of fat as a source of energy, and that has distinct health benefits. And if your goal is performance, you should include some training at or near your lactate threshold. Remember, training must be specific to its intended purpose if you are to achieve optimal results.

Intensity is important, but excessive emphasis on intensity can take the joy out of regular activity. Athletes don't train hard every day, and you shouldn't either. That is why I encourage you to move beyond the objective approach of heart rates and training zones to the subjective, where you utilize perceived exertion and listen to your body. Adopt the active life gradually, enjoying the experience, the adaptations, and the amazing results.

7

Aerobic Fitness Programs

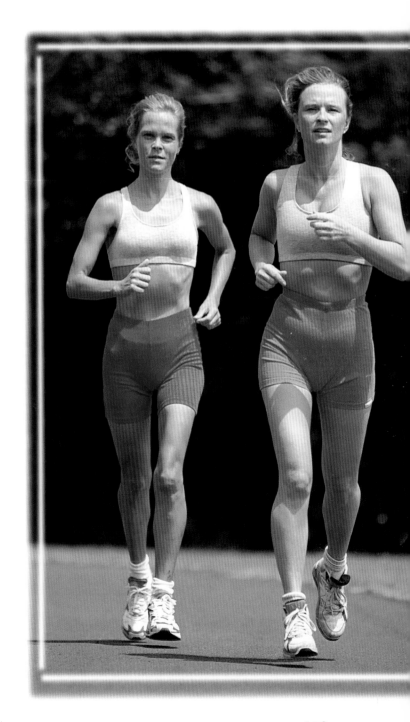

"You will never find time for anything. If you want time you must make it."

Charles Buxton

113

People often tell me they would like to become more fit but they just haven't got the time. I tell them how others make time for regular exercise, including the last five U.S. presidents and many other busy people. The time has come for you to make time for regular fitness training. This chapter provides training tips, training programs, and other information you'll need to make training safe, enjoyable, and effective. The programs in this chapter have been proven to be cost-effective, providing maximum benefit for the time invested.

■ This chapter will help you

- understand how to make training safe and enjoyable;
- apply your aerobic fitness prescription via
  - walk-jog-run programs,
  - cycling or swimming programs, or
  - advanced aerobic training;
- select alternative ways to remain active and fit; and
- deal with common exercise problems.

Training Tips

We'll begin with walking and running as modes of exercise because, for the time and cost, they provide a great training stimulus. Intensity and duration are easy to control, and the activities can be done at any time, in almost any weather, with little investment in equipment. The equipment is light and easily transported on vacation or business trips. You can participate alone or in a group and can continue throughout life. A recent study of 72,488 female nurses found that brisk walking was inversely associated with the risk of heart disease; the relative risk declined as the amount of walking increased (Manson et al. 1999). The benefits were similar to those achieved with other forms of vigorous exercise, such as running. For these reasons and more, walking and running are fine ways to achieve and maintain aerobic fitness and its benefits.

What to Wear

Nothing is more important to your enjoyment than comfortable shoes, so don't economize when you purchase footwear. Go to a reputable sporting goods dealer and seek advice from a knowledgeable salesperson. Avoid sale shoes at discount outlets unless you know something about the product. Buy a training shoe, not one built for competition. A firm, thick sole; good arch support; and a well-padded heel are essential. The sole should be firm but not terribly difficult to flex. A firm heel counter is also important. If blisters are a problem, try tube socks, a thin sock under a heavier one, or petroleum jelly on potential hot spots.

Walking and jogging don't require fancy clothing. Nylon or cotton shorts and a T-shirt are adequate in summer. For winter, a jogging suit serves until temperatures fall below 20 degrees Fahrenheit (minus 7 degrees Celsius). Some runners prefer tights. Just remember that layers of lighter clothing are preferable to a single heavy garment. Add gloves and a knit cap in colder temperatures. When the wind blows, a thin windbreaker helps reduce heat loss. A cap is important in cold weather because you lose a great deal of heat from your head. When it is really cold, you can wear tights and wind pants. Many runners continue in subzero

A cap is important in cold weather because you lose a great deal of heat from your head.

temperatures, which is safe provided you are properly clothed, warmed up, and sensitive to the signs of wind chill and frostbite (see chapter 17). For longer winter outings, I prefer to use polypropylene underwear to wick perspiration away from the skin, thereby avoiding rapid cooling. Add a pile vest and a windbreaker, and you are ready to go.

Technique

An upright posture conserves energy. Run or walk with your back comfortably straight, your head up, and your shoulders relaxed. When jogging, bend your arms, hold your hands in a comfortable position, and keep arm swing to a minimum. Pumping action will increase with more speed. Swing your legs freely from the hip with no attempt to overstride. Studies show that the stride that feels best is usually the most efficient as well.

I recommend the *heel-to-toe* footstrike for most new runners. It is the least tiring, and most distance runners use it. Land lightly on the heel, and roll forward to push off the ball of the foot. For faster running employ a slight forward lean, more knee lift, a quick and forceful push-off, and more arm action. Check your shoes after several weeks of running; the outer border of the heel will show some wear if you are using the correct footstrike.

Time of Day

Exercise whenever it suits your fancy. Some people prefer to work out before breakfast, others during the lunch hour or after work. A few night owls brave the dark in their quest for fitness; the run and shower help them sleep. Avoid vigorous exercise (except walking, cycling, or cross-country skiing) for one to two hours after a meal, when the digestive system requires an adequate blood supply. I like to run during the lunch hour. If I go out with a problem, I often come back with a solution.

Unless you need time alone, consider training with a partner. Find one with similar abilities, interests, and goals, and you aren't likely to miss your workout.

Where to Walk or Run

Avoid hard surfaces for the first weeks of training. Walk or run in the park, on playing fields, on a golf course, or on a running track. Then you'll be ready to try the back roads or trails in your area. Varying your routes will help you maintain interest. When the weather prohibits outdoor exercise, try a mall, YMCA, or school gym, or choose an exercise supplement you can do at home, such as running in place or skipping rope. I suggest other aerobic alternatives later in this chapter.

Sample Aerobic Fitness Programs

Your fitness prescription gives you the freedom to tailor a fitness program to meet your specific needs. You have a wide choice of exercises and also many options in the length of time you want to exercise and the intensity of that activity. Some people prefer a more detailed, step-by-step approach. For this reason, I've included some walk-jog-run programs.

I'll describe programs for three levels of ability: a starter program for those in low-fitness categories (aerobic fitness score under 35 ml/kg · min), an intermediate program (35 to 45), and one for those in high-fitness categories (45 or better). The starter program was prepared by the President's Council on Physical Fitness and Sport and appears in the booklet "An Introduction to Physical Fitness."

Starter Programs (Walk-Jog-Run)

Take the walk test to determine your exercise level.

Walk Test

The object of this test is to determine how many minutes (up to 10) you can walk at a brisk pace, on a level surface, without undue difficulty or discomfort.

If you can't walk for 5 minutes, begin with the *red* walking program. If you can walk more than 5 minutes, but less than 10, begin with the third week of the *red* walking program. If you can walk for the full 10 minutes but are somewhat tired and sore as a result, start with the *white* walk-jog program. If you can breeze through the full 10 minutes, you're ready for bigger things. Wait until the next day and take the 10-minute walk-jog test.

Walk-Jog Test

In this test you alternately walk 50 steps (left foot strikes the ground 25 times) and jog 50 steps for a total of 10 minutes. Walk at the rate of 120 steps per minute (left foot strikes the ground at 1-second intervals). Jog at the rate of 144 steps per minute (left foot strikes the ground 18 times every 15 seconds).

If you can't complete the 10-minute test, begin at the third week of the *white* program. If you can complete the 10-minute test but are tired and winded as a result, start with the last week of the *white* program before moving to the *blue* program. If you can perform the 10-minute walk-jog test without difficulty, start with the *blue* program.

Red Walking Program

Start with this program, doing each activity every other day at first (see figure 7.1). The first week you'll walk at a brisk pace for five minutes, or for a shorter time if you become uncomfortably tired. Walk slowly or rest for three minutes. Then walk briskly again for five minutes or until you become uncomfortably tired. The second week of the program is the same, but increase your pace as soon as you can walk five minutes without soreness or fatigue. During the third week of the program you'll increase your brisk walking to eight minutes. Increase your pace in the fourth week. When you've completed week 4 of the red program, begin at week 1 of the white program.

White Walk-Jog Program

In this program you'll begin by walking at a brisk pace for 10 minutes, or for a shorter time if you become uncomfortably tired (see figure 7.2). After a slow walk or rest you'll resume the brisk pace. The second week will increase the amount of time spent walking at a brisk pace; the third and fourth weeks will incorporate jogging short distances. Do each activity four times a week. When you've completed week 4 of the white program, begin week 1 of the blue program.

Blue Jogging Program

In this program you'll increase the amount of time spent jogging each week (see figure 7.3). Do each activity five times a week, as indicated.

Week	Sunday	Monday	Tuesday	Wednesday	Thursday	Friday	Saturday
1	Brisk walk 5 min Slow walk/ rest 3 min Brisk walk 5 min		Brisk walk 5 min Slow walk/ rest 3 min Brisk walk 5 min		Brisk walk 5 min Slow walk/ rest 3 min Brisk walk 5 min		Brisk walk 5 min Slow walk/ rest 3 min Brisk walk 5 min
2		Brisk walk 5 min Slow walk/ rest 3 min Brisk walk 5 min		Brisk walk 5 min Slow walk/ rest 3 min Brisk walk 5 min		Brisk walk 5 min Slow walk/ rest 3 min Brisk walk 5 min	
3	Brisk walk 8 min Slow walk/ rest 3 min Brisk walk 8 min		Brisk walk 8 min Slow walk/ rest 3 min Brisk walk 8 min		Brisk walk 8 min Slow walk/ rest 3 min Brisk walk 8 min		Brisk walk 8 min Slow walk/ rest 3 min Brisk walk 8 min
4		Brisk walk 8 min Slow walk/ rest 3 min Brisk walk 8 min		Brisk walk 8 min Slow walk/ rest 3 min Brisk walk 8 min		Brisk walk 8 min Slow walk/ rest 3 min Brisk walk 8 min	

Figure 7.1   Red walking program.

Intermediate Jog-Run Program

If you've followed the starter program or are already reasonably active, you're ready for the intermediate program (see figure 7.4). You're able to jog 1 mile (1.6 kilometers) slowly without undue fatigue, rest two minutes, and do it again. Your sessions consume about 250 calories.

You're ready to increase both the intensity and the duration of your runs. You'll be using the heart rate training zone for those of medium fitness (35 to 45 ml/kg · min). You'll begin jogging 1 mile (1.6 kilometers) in 12 minutes, and when you finish this program you may be able to complete 3 miles (4.8 kilometers) or more at a pace approaching 8 minutes per mile. Each week's program includes three phases—the basic workout, longer runs (overdistance), and shorter runs (underdistance). If a week's program seems too easy, move ahead; if it seems too hard, move back a week or two. On most of the days, you'll jog in intervals and walk to recover. For example, on Tuesday of the first week, begin by jogging .25 to .5 mile (.4 to .8 kilometer) slowly. Then try to jog .5 mile in 5 minutes 30 seconds,

Week	Sunday	Monday	Tuesday	Wednesday	Thursday	Friday	Saturday
1	Brisk walk 10 min Slow walk/rest 3 min Brisk walk 10 min	Brisk walk 10 min Slow walk/rest 3 min Brisk walk 10 min		Brisk walk 10 min Slow walk/rest 3 min Brisk walk 10 min		Brisk walk 10 min Slow walk/rest 3 min Brisk walk 10 min	
2	Brisk walk 15 min Slow walk/rest 3 min Brisk walk 10 min		Brisk walk 15 min Slow walk/rest 3 min Brisk walk 10 min		Brisk walk 15 min Slow walk/rest 3 min Brisk walk 15 min		Brisk walk 15 min Slow walk/rest 3 min Brisk walk 15 min
3	Jog 10 s (25 yd) Walk 1 min (100 yd) 12x		Jog 10 s (25 yd) Walk 1 min (100 yd) 12x		Jog 10 s (25 yd) Walk 1 min (100 yd) 12x		Jog 10 s (25 yd) Walk 1 min (100 yd) 12x
4		Jog 20 s (50 yd) Walk 1 min (100 yd) 12x		Jog 20 s (50 yd) Walk 1 min (100 yd) 12x		Jog 20 s (50 yd) Walk 1 min (100 yd) 12x	Jog 20 s (50 yd) Walk 1 min (100 yd) 12x

Figure 7.2 White walk-jog program.

walk to recover, and repeat. Next, jog .25 mile in 2 minutes 45 seconds, walk to recover, and repeat three times. Finally, jog .25 to .5 mile as in the beginning of the workout. On Thursday, jog 1 mile in 12 minutes, walk to recover, and repeat. Table 7.1 on page 123 is a pace guide for gauging your speed over various distances. Remember to warm up and cool down as part of every exercise session.

Advanced Aerobic Training

This section is for the well-trained individual. I'll provide some suggestions for advanced training, but keep in mind that there is no single way to train. If you enjoy underdistance training, by all means use it. If you find that you prefer overdistance, use that approach.

Simply pick up the pace as you approach the end of a long run, and you'll receive an optimal training stimulus. Moreover, because the speed work is limited to a short span near the end of the run, discomfort is brief.

Consider the following suggestions:

- Always warm up before your run.
- Use the high-fitness heart rate training zone.

Week	Sunday	Monday	Tuesday	Wednesday	Thursday	Friday	Saturday
1	Jog 40 s (100 yd) Walk 1 min (100 yd) 9x	Jog 40 s (100 yd) Walk 1 min (100 yd) 9x		Jog 40 s (100 yd) Walk 1 min (100 yd) 9x	Jog 40 s (100 yd) Walk 1 min (100 yd) 9x		Jog 40 s (100 yd) Walk 1 min (100 yd) 9x
2	Jog 1 min (150 yd) Walk 1 min (100 yd) 8x	Jog 1 min (150 yd) Walk 1 min (100 yd) 8x	Jog 1 min (150 yd) Walk 1 min (100 yd) 8x		Jog 1 min (150 yd) Walk 1 min (100 yd) 8x	Jog 1 min (150 yd) Walk 1 min (100 yd) 8x	
3	Jog 2 min (300 yd) Walk 1 min (100 yd) 6x	Jog 2 min (300 yd) Walk 1 min (100 yd) 6x		Jog 2 min (300 yd) Walk 1 min (100 yd) 6x	Jog 2 min (300 yd) Walk 1 min (100 yd) 6x		Jog 2 min (300 yd) Walk 1 min (100 yd) 6x
4	Jog 4 min (600 yd) Walk 1 min (100 yd) 4x		Jog 4 min (600 yd) Walk 1 min (100 yd) 4x	Jog 4 min (600 yd) Walk 1 min (100 yd) 4x		Jog 4 min (600 yd) Walk 1 min (100 yd) 4x	Jog 4 min (600 yd) Walk 1 min (100 yd) 4x
5	Jog 6 min (900 yd) Walk 1 min (100 yd) 3x	Jog 6 min (900 yd) Walk 1 min (100 yd) 3x		Jog 6 min (900 yd) Walk 1 min (100 yd) 3x	Jog 6 min (900 yd) Walk 1 min (100 yd) 3x		Jog 6 min (900 yd) Walk 1 min (100 yd) 3x
6	Jog 8 min (1,200 yd) Walk 2 min (200 yd) 2x		Jog 8 min (1,200 yd) Walk 2 min (200 yd) 2x	Jog 8 min (1,200 yd) Walk 2 min (200 yd) 2x		Jog 8 min (1,200 yd) Walk 2 min (200 yd) 2x	Jog 8 min (1,200 yd) Walk 2 min (200 yd) 2x
7	Jog 10 min (1,500 yd) Walk 2 min (200 yd) 2x	Jog 10 min (1,500 yd) Walk 2 min (200 yd) 2x		Jog 10 min (1,500 yd) Walk 2 min (200 yd) 2x	Jog 10 min (1,500 yd) Walk 2 min (200 yd) 2x		Jog 10 min (1,500 yd) Walk 2 min (200 yd) 2x
8	Jog 12 min (1,760 yd) Walk 2 min (200 yd) 2x		Jog 12 min (1,760 yd) Walk 2 min (200 yd) 2x	Jog 12 min (1,760 yd) Walk 2 min (200 yd) 2x		Jog 12 min (1,760 yd) Walk 2 min (200 yd) 2x	Jog 12 min (1,760 yd) Walk 2 min (200 yd) 2x

Figure 7.3 Blue jogging program.

Week	Monday	Tuesday	Wednesday	Thursday	Friday	Saturday/ Sunday
1	1 mi (12 min) Walk 2x	1/4-1/2 mi slow 2 x 1/2 mi (5.30 min) 4 x 1/4 mi (2.45 min) 1/4-1/2 mi jog	2 mi slow jog	1 mi (12 min) Walk 2x	1/4-1/2 mi slow 2 x 1/2 mi (5.30 min) 4 x 1/4 mi (2.45 min) 1/4-1/2 mi jog	2 mi slow jog
2	1 mi (11 min) Walk 2x	1/4-1/2 mi slow 1/2 mi (5 min) 2 x 1/4 mi (2.30 min) 2 x 1/4 mi (2.45 min) 4 x 220 yd (1.20 min) 1/4-1/2 mi slow	2 1/4 mi slow jog	1 mi (11 min) Walk 2x	1/4-1/2 mi slow 1/2 mi (5 min) 2 x 1/4 mi (2.30 min) 2 x 1/4 mi (2.45 min) 4 x 220 yd (1.20 min) 1/4-1/2 mi slow	2 1/4 mi slow jog
3	1 mi (10.30 min) Walk 2x	1/4-1/2 mi slow 1/2 mi (4.45 min) 4 x 1/4 mi (2.30 min) 4 x 220 yd (1.10 min) 4 x 100 yd (0.30 min) 1/4-1/2 mi slow	2 1/2 mi slow jog	1 mi (10.30 min) Walk 2x	1/4-1/2 mi slow 1/2 mi (4.45 min) 4 x 1/4 mi (2.30 min) 4 x 220 yd (1.10 min) 4 x 100 yd (0.30 min) 1/4-1/2 mi slow	2 1/2 mi slow jog
4	1 mi (10 min) Walk 2x	1/4-1/2 mi slow 2 x 1/2 mi (4.45 min) 4 x 1/4 mi (2.20 min) 4 x 220 yd (1 min) 1/4-1/2 mi slow	2 3/4 mi slow jog	1 mi (10 min) Walk 2x	1/4-1/2 mi slow 2 x 1/2 mi (4.45 min) 4 x 1/4 mi (2.20 min) 4 x 220 yd (1 min) 1/4-1/2 mi slow	2 3/4 mi slow jog

Figure 7.4 Intermediate jog-run program. Times are given in minutes and seconds (e.g., 2.45 min is 2 minutes and 45 seconds).

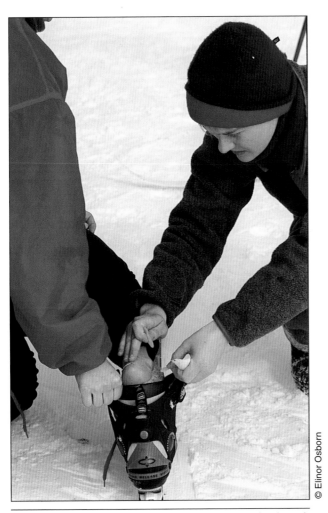

© Elinor Osborn

Prevention is the most effective way to deal with exercise problems.

but don't stop there. Find out why it hurts (e.g., old shoes) and correct the problem once and for all.

Common Problems

You can deal with many of the problems that threaten to diminish your enjoyment of training.

Blisters

Blisters are minor burns caused by friction. You can prevent them by using properly fitted shoes, appropriate socks (double-layer or tube socks), and a lubricant (e.g., petroleum jelly) on potential hot spots. At the first hint of a blister, cover the area with moleskin or a large bandage. Advanced cases can be treated with a sterilized hollow needle. Release the fluid, treat with an antiseptic, circle the area with a foam rubber donut, and go back to work. Keep a blister prevention kit in your locker or gym bag, and always carry the kit on hiking trips.

Muscle Soreness

Delayed onset muscle soreness (DOMS) develops about 24 hours after a new or more vigorous exercise. It occurs in the muscles involved and may be due to microscopic tears in the muscle or connective tissue, to swelling, or to localized contractions of muscle fibers. You can minimize the soreness by phasing into a sport gradually. Mild stretching and warming up make subsequent activity less painful. Massage seems to reduce the discomfort. The good news is that DOMS is a temporary inconvenience that inoculates you from further discomfort—at least until you start a new sport.

Muscle Cramps

A cramp is a powerful involuntary contraction that results when the muscle refuses to relax. Normally, the nervous system tells muscles when to contract and when to relax, but when the normal control fails, the result can be painful. Immediate relief comes when the cramped muscle is stretched and massaged. However, that does not remove the underlying cause of the involuntary contraction. Salt and calcium are involved in the chemistry of contraction and relaxation. Hot temperatures and dehydration seem to predispose muscles to cramps. Attend to fluid and electrolyte replacement during activity in hot weather.

Bone Bruises

Hikers and joggers sometimes get painful bruises on the soles of their feet. You can avoid such bruises with careful foot placement and quality footwear. Cushioned inner soles and gel- or air-sole shoes can aid in reducing the repetitive shocks that lead to bruises. A bad bruise can last for weeks. Ice may lessen discomfort, and padding may allow some activity. When bruises occur, examine your shoes; it may be time to replace them.

Ankle Problems

Treatment for a sprained ankle involves RICES (see below). Ice the ankle immediately, preferably in a bucket of ice water. Ice several times a day, and in between, rest and elevate the ankle. Use a wrap to stabilize and maintain compression. When possible, use high-top shoes to prevent ankle problems. Tape or lace-on supports may allow some activity after the swelling subsides.

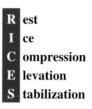

R est
I ce
C ompression
E levation
S tabilization

Calf or Achilles Tendon Injuries

A pulling sensation in the calf or Achilles tendon cannot be ignored. Treat minor pulls with rest, ice, and gel heel cups. Return to activity cautiously; a serious pull can take weeks to heal. Prevent calf or Achilles problems with adequate stretching, good footwear, and a gradual warm-up.

Shinsplints

Pain on the front portion of the shinbones is known as shinsplints. It can be caused by inflammation of the tibialis anterior muscle, its membrane, or the bone it attaches to, or a spasm of the inflamed muscle. Rest, compression wraps, deep massage (toward heart), ultrasound, and anti-inflammatory drugs (e.g., ibuprofen) provide some relief. Prevention involves gradual adjustment to training, avoidance of hard running surfaces, occasional reversal of direction when running on a curved track, use of the heel-to-toe footstrike, resistance exercises, and stretching.

Knee Problems

Research suggests that running doesn't harm healthy knees. Unfortunately, many of us run on less than healthy knees, knees already afflicted with osteoarthritis. My high school football injury left me with an arthritic knee. Surprisingly, I have been able to continue running with the help of several aids. I do weight training to maintain muscle strength in stabilizing thigh and hamstring muscles. I ride a bike to add strength and endurance without trauma. And I take a nonsteroidal anti-inflammatory drug (NSAID) such as aspirin or ibuprofen to quiet inflammation and discomfort in the degenerative joint. Overuse (e.g., a long hike or run) calls for a bit more of the NSAID, ice, and compression until things cool down.

If you experience runner's knee or some other problem, correct the cause while you treat the symptom. Try new shoes or arch supports. Alternate between two pairs of shoes if you run a lot, one with padding for sore feet and the other with a flexible sole for sore legs. If these ideas don't help, consult an athletic trainer, or a podiatrist who specializes in sports medicine. Specialists may recommend foot supports (orthotics) to help your problem. These plastic inserts can correct pronation and reduce some knee pain.

Stitch

The side pain called a stitch, usually blamed on food or fluid in the digestive system, may be due to tugging of ligaments that attach the gut to the diaphragm. A treadmill study induced the stitch by giving the subjects a drink, then used several techniques to reduce their discomfort. Bending forward while tightening the abdominal muscles, exhaling through pursed lips, or tightening a belt around the waist were dramatically effective treatments. The authors suggested that the results were consistent with a ligamentous origin for the stitch (Plunkett and Hopkins 1995).

Overuse Syndromes

If you go too far or too fast too soon, if you forget to stretch or warm up, if you have muscle imbalances, if one leg is shorter than the other, or if you have weak feet, you are bound to have overuse problems now and then. Use ice for all acute strains and sprains. Keep an ice "popsicle" in the freezer and use it several times a day to reduce inflammation and hasten recovery (tape a tongue depressor upright in a cup of water and put it in the freezer). Rub the problem area with ice until it becomes numb. You'll be amazed by your rapid return to activity.

NSAIDs

I have found that the careful use of the nonsteroidal anti-inflammatory drugs (NSAIDs) aspirin and ibuprofen helps minimize many nagging problems and some big ones. With a doctor's advice I started taking aspirin more than 25 years ago to quiet a painful knee. In recent years we have learned that one pill a day reduces blood clotting and the risks of heart attacks. Aspirin also reduces the little strokes (transient ischemic attacks) that become more prevalent with age. Ibuprofen, which I take for muscle and joint pain, has been associated with a lower risk of Alzheimer's disease. Both of these drugs cause stomach irritation, and some people are allergic to aspirin. But in small doses, taken with food to minimize stomach irritation, aspirin and ibuprofen offer amazing relief for the price.

Aspirin reduces pain and inflammation by inhibiting the production of cell hormones called prostaglandins. Exercise can cause prostaglandin production, which may lead to soreness. A single NSAID before exercise can reduce the need for larger doses afterward. Judicious use of NSAIDs keeps many aging athletes active long after others have given up.

Exercise Hazards

Regular moderate physical activity is an established aid to health, fitness, weight control, and longevity. The term *regular* is understood by all, but the concept of *moderate* requires definition. Moderate exercise for an athlete may be hazardous for the sedentary adult. Moderate exercise can be defined as a level likely to bring about improved fitness without exposing the individual to the hazards of strenuous effort. The heart rate training zone is one guide to moderate exercise, as is perceived exertion or the talk test. If you can carry on a conversation during exercise, the level is not too intense.

Sudden Vigorous Exercise

Failure to warm up before vigorous exercise can result in electrocardiogram abnormalities, regardless of the fitness or age of the subjects. Dr. Jerry Barnard found such abnormalities in 31 of 44 apparently healthy firemen tested on a vigorous treadmill test. The findings indicated inadequate blood flow in the coronary arteries and lack of oxygen to the heart. A warm-up consisting of a five-minute jog prevented the problems (Barnard et al. 1972). It appears that athletes aren't the only ones who need to warm up; anyone performing vigorous work or exercise can benefit. Calisthenic warm-ups are common among factory workers in Europe and Japan, but they are less common in the United States. Though most workers can and should warm up, it is hard to see, for example, how law enforcement officers can do so before chasing a suspect. For this reason they should do all they can to keep fit and healthy.

Stressful Exercise

Stress is something that the individual perceives as a threat. The body reacts to the threat by secreting a group of hormones that assist the mobilization of energy and prepare the body for combat or retreat (fight or flight). The body does not differentiate between physical and mental threats; it reacts similarly to each. An important exam may be stressful to a medical student, or a canoe trip could be stressful to a nonswimmer. Stress accelerates clotting time of the blood, which is good for a soldier in battle or a boxer in the ring, but bad for an adult with atherosclerosis, where a clot could block the flow of blood to the heart. Though exercise is not inherently stressful, studies indicate that unfamiliar, exhausting, and competitive exercise can be stressful for some people.

Unfamiliar Exercise

A person's first skiing or mountain climbing experience may be stressful, but the stress diminishes as skill and confidence grow. We found faster clotting time on a subject's first treadmill test but normal clotting after weeks of experience, when the test was no longer perceived as a threat (Whiddon, Sharkey, and Steadman 1969). Early experiences in unfamiliar or threatening exercise situations, such as white-water kayaking, should be preceded with less-threatening introductions, such as a session in a pool.

Exhausting Exercise

In experiments on dogs, a Japanese researcher found that exhaustion could be stressful (Suzuki 1967). The animals were taken for runs of various intensities and durations by a bike-riding attendant. Only exhausting runs increased the secretion of stress hormones. The researcher concluded that nonexhausting exercise need not be stressful. Of course, it is possible that the stress associated with exhaustion was due, at least in part, by the dogs' fear of being left behind.

Competitive Exercise

Years ago, researchers at Harvard University studied the stress responses to various types of competition in rowers. Crew members did not perceive the strenuous effort of practice as a threat, but they did demonstrate increased hormone levels after either a time trial or a competitive race. The nonexercising coxswain also exhibited a stress response after the competitive event. The researchers concluded that exercise, by itself, was not stressful, but the excitement of competition did elicit the response, with or without exertion (Hill, Goetz, and Fox 1956).

The hormones of the stress response are required for the full mobilization of resources and the maximal performance of the athlete. I would never suggest that healthy men or women should avoid the excitement of unfamiliar, exhausting, or competitive sport or activity. However, previously inactive individuals should prepare for participation with training and gradual exposure to the stress involved. In time, the unfamiliar becomes familiar, training reduces exhaustion, and the athlete within learns to cope with the physical and psychological requirements of competition.

Indeed, adults regularly engage in stressful activities. For many, the excitement of sport keeps them active. Those who thrive on challenge, excitement, or exhaustion do so after long periods of preparation. Aging athletes continue to practice and train in order to remain competitive. If you want to become involved in competitive tennis, distance running, or mountain climbing, give yourself time to adjust to the demands. Improve your fitness and skill as you prepare for your first exposure. Set reasonable goals and never take the results too seriously.

For many, the excitement of sport keeps them active.

Summary

This chapter has presented training tips; walking, running, and other training programs; aerobic alternatives; and advice on how to handle some common problems. You are welcome to adopt one of the programs or to use your aerobic prescription and fashion your own approach. I'm often amazed by the ingenious and personal approaches that some folks devise—such as the retired zoology professor who regularly climbs the mountain behind our campus, both for exercise and to observe the flora and fauna. Years ago, before it was in vogue, he decided to use ski poles to exercise his arms while lowering the load on his legs. The poles become even more important on the return trip, relieving stress on his knees during the steep descent. His creative adaptation has extended his range and saved his knees for many more years of enjoyable outdoor exercise. Recently I've added a telescoping ski pole to my hiking and backpacking gear, and I wonder why I didn't do it years ago.

An addition to my personal program has been regular attention to muscular fitness. It too has helped me up and over many a steep trail. Let's see how it can help you.

PART III

Muscular Fitness

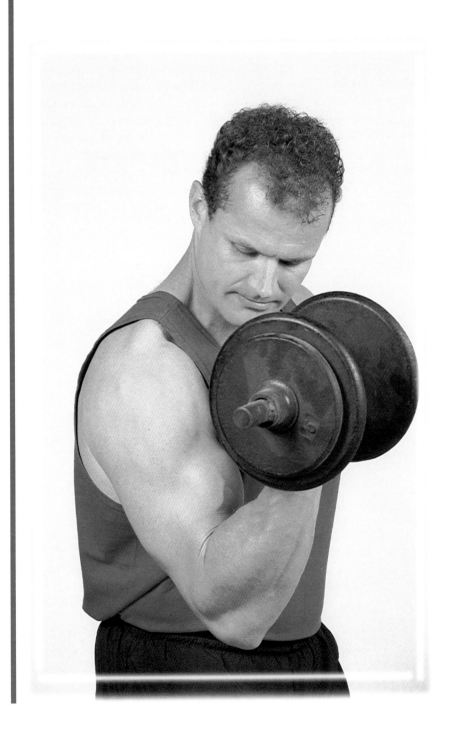

Not too many years ago, muscular fitness occupied an awkward position on the fringe of the fitness movement. We recognized its contributions to performance in sport and some forms of work, but we lacked conclusive evidence linking muscular fitness with health and the quality of life. That has now changed, and we can say with confidence that both aerobic and muscular fitness contribute substantially to health. Muscular fitness training increases muscle mass, the furnace that burns fat. Exercises that improve muscular fitness help you avoid the crippling bone demineralization known as osteoporosis. Attention to muscular fitness is essential if you are to avoid the low back problems and repetitive motion injuries that plague millions of Americans. And continued participation insures the capacity for independence and mobility in your postretirement years.

The essential components of muscular fitness are strength, muscular endurance, and flexibility. Other important components include power, speed, agility, and balance. With most physiologic capabilities, you either use them or lose them, and that is certainly true for muscular fitness. Strength, endurance, flexibility, power, agility, and balance all decline with age. However, the rate of decline is much slower for those who remain active. And recent studies show that we have the capability to build strength even into our 90s (Fiatarone et al. 1994)!

But don't wait until you are 90 to experience the pleasures and rewards of muscular fitness. Begin now, and you will soon notice that tasks are easier, your muscles are firmer, your tummy is flatter, and you just feel better about yourself and life in general.

because of elastic recoil and a favorable alignment of contractile proteins); the rested muscle exerts more force than a fatigued one; and mechanical factors conspire to magnify force or speed. Several other factors, including gender, age, fiber type, and training deserve attention.

Gender

Until 12 to 14 years of age, boys are not much stronger than girls. Thereafter, the average male gains an advantage that persists throughout life. Is the difference due to the increase in the male hormone testosterone at puberty? Perhaps; the average male has 10 times the testosterone found in the average female. Testosterone is an anabolic (growth-inducing) steroid that helps muscles get larger. College women have 50 to 60 percent of the arm and shoulder strength and 70 percent of the leg strength of their male counterparts. But a relationship doesn't imply cause and effect. The relationship of strength and testosterone might also be related to a third factor. For example, the hormone may make men more aggressive and willing to train harder.

Consider another confounding possibility: body fat. Young women average twice the percentage of fat as men (25 percent versus 12.5 percent). When you look at strength per unit of lean body weight (body weight minus fat weight), women have slightly stronger legs, whereas arm strength remains 30 percent below the men's values. Wilmore (1983) suggests that because women use their legs as men do (walking, climbing stairs, bicycling), their leg muscles are similar in strength. Because fewer women use their arms in heavy work or sport, their strength lags behind in this area. Thus it may be a mistake to judge women the weaker sex. As more women engage in upper body strength training for sport or occupational purposes (police, fire fighting, construction), their strength will certainly come closer to that of men.

However, muscle size and strength do go together for both genders, and the average male is larger than the average female. Most studies indicate a force of four to six kilograms per square centimeter of muscle girth. To estimate muscle girth in the upper arm, you should measure subcutaneous fat and bone size as well, because they will be part of the total circumference. All other things being equal, the larger muscle is the stronger one, but not necessarily the most successful in work or sport.

Age

Strength reaches a peak in the early 20s and declines slowly until about age 60. Thereafter the rate of decline usually accelerates, but it doesn't have to. When strength is used, it hardly declines at all, even into the 60s. Champion weight lifters have achieved personal records in their 40s. Auto mechanics retain grip strength into their 60s. Training before puberty leads to improvements that are mostly due to changes in the nervous system (neurogenic factors include reduced inhibitions and learning how to exert force). Training after puberty combines nervous system changes with changes in the muscle tissue (myogenic changes). Because testosterone levels decline in old age, many physiologists thought that senior citizens would be limited to neurogenic changes when they engaged in strength training. However, a study of very elderly people (72 to 98 years) has shown that resistance training leads to increased strength, muscle mass, and mobility (Fiatarone et al. 1994). Training at any age maintains or improves strength, especially when the diet is adequate. We'll say more about both later on.

Training at any age maintains or improves strength, especially when the diet is adequate.

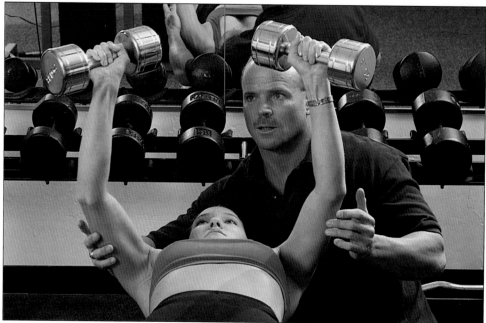

Both men and women benefit from strength training.

Muscle Fiber Types

Earlier I noted the presence of two fiber types, slow-twitch and fast-twitch. The larger, faster-contracting fast-twitch fibers have a greater potential for the development of tension. Individuals with a higher percentage of fast-twitch fibers have a greater potential for force development. Studies of human muscle tissue reveal that weight lifters have twice the area of fast-twitch fibers as nonlifters. The size can be attributed to heredity and to training. The effect of strength training on muscle fiber types has yet to be completely resolved; current evidence indicates that both types grow larger with training, but growth of the fast fibers is more pronounced. Strength training improves the capabilities of both types but doesn't seem to change one type into another.

Types of Strength

Strength can be measured and developed in several ways, each of which is highly specific. How the strength will be used should dictate the mode of training and testing.

Dynamic Strength

Also called *isotonic,* dynamic strength is defined as the maximal weight that can be lifted one time. This is actually a measure of strength at the hardest part of the lift, usually the beginning. Because the mechanical advantage of your muscle-lever system changes, a lift such as a forearm curl becomes easier after you overcome the initial resistance and angle of pull. Dynamic strength measurements are related to performance in sport and work. Weightlifting with machines or free weights is the common form of isotonic training. (*Iso* means "same," *tonic* means "tone"; so *isotonic* means "same tone.")

Static Strength

The measure of static strength is achieved when one exerts maximal force against an immovable object. Also called *isometric* strength, it is specific to the angle at which it was trained. It doesn't necessarily reflect dynamic strength or strength throughout the range of motion. You train by exerting near maximum force against an immovable object. (*Metric* means "length"; *isometric* means "same length"—the muscle doesn't change length appreciably during the contraction.)

Isokinetic Strength

Isokinetic strength is measured with an expensive electronic or hydraulic apparatus. It allows the exertion of maximal force throughout the range of motion, as well as the control of the speed of contraction. Though such devices have become popular testing aids, it is not yet clear to what extent strength throughout the range of motion is related to performance. (*Kinetic* means "motion" or "speed"; *isokinetic* means "same speed.")

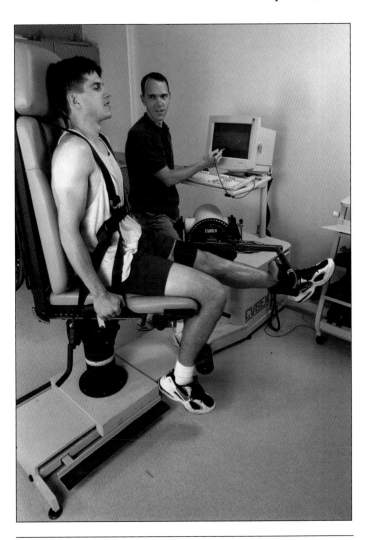

Figure 8.2 Sports medicine specialists test knee extension and flexion strength, power, and endurance and use isokinetic devices to rehabilitate athletes following knee surgery.

A number of sophisticated devices are available for the isokinetic measurement of muscle force and power. Sports medicine specialists test knee extension and flexion strength, power, and endurance and use isokinetic devices to rehabilitate athletes following knee surgery. Variable and accommodating resistance devices are used to strengthen muscles and to prevent injuries (figures 8.2 and 8.3).

Examples of these devices include *variable resistance* (resistance varies with speed of contraction) and *accommodating resistance* (resistance accommodates to available force). Though each type of apparatus has some interesting features, no method or system has proven superior in the development of strength in subjects with little previous muscular fitness training. More experienced lifters will use the method suited to and specific for the task or activity. Athletes may use free weights, isokinetic machines, and even isometric contractions in an effort to improve performance. Strength is specific to the method of training, to the speed of contractions, and to the angle employed in training. Therefore, the method of testing should be specific to the mode of training if you want to accurately assess the effects of training. In other words, don't use a static strength test to reflect changes from dynamic strength training or vice versa.

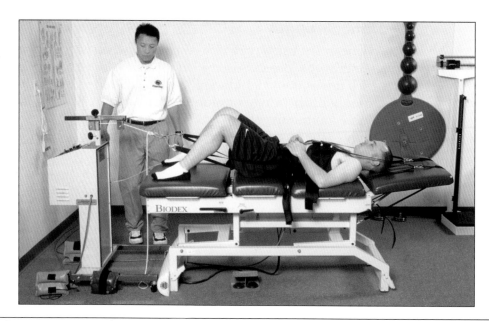

Figure 8.3 New devices are changing the way back problems are evaluated and treated.

Muscular Endurance

Muscular endurance is essential for success in many work and sport activities.

Muscular endurance means the ability to persist. It is defined and measured as the repetition of submaximal contractions or submaximal holding time (isometric endurance). Muscular endurance is essential for success in many work and sport activities. Once you have the strength to perform a repetitive task, additional improvement in performance will depend on muscular endurance, the ability to persist. As mentioned earlier, stronger fast-twitch fibers fatigue more readily. Thus endurance and strength are not highly related, except when a very heavy load is used in an endurance test.

Endurance?

I use the term *muscular endurance* to differentiate it from other uses of the term. It is possible to develop considerable endurance in small muscles, such as the finger flexors used by a pianist or barber, without any noticeable effect on the heart or respiratory systems. My barber has great endurance in the muscles of his fingers, but his aerobic fitness is poor. Muscular endurance resides in metabolic adaptations and neuromuscular efficiency of the fibers used in the activity.

Endurance and Strength

Let's spend a moment contrasting endurance and strength, which are really quite different in physiological terms. Endurance is achieved by repetitive contractions of muscle fibers. Repetitive contractions require a continuous supply of energy, and muscle fibers with aerobic (oxidative) capabilities (slow oxidative, fast oxidative glycolytic) are suited to the job. The repetitive contractions enhance aerobic enzymes, mitochondria, and the fuels needed for repetitive contractions.

Strength comes from lifting heavy loads a few times. As we have said, the effects of strength training are most noticeable in fast-twitch fibers. Training effects include increases in contractile proteins (actin and myosin) and tougher connec-

9
Benefits of Muscular Fitness

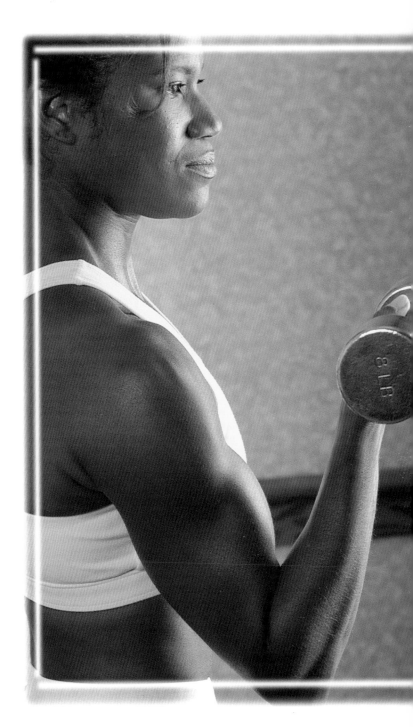

". . . power waits upon
him who earns it."

John Burroughs

How does training lead to changes in muscle fibers? How does a muscle fiber know the difference between strength and endurance training? Part of the answer to these questions is related to the training stimulus, the characteristic of training that leads to specific adaptations. Strength improves when sufficient *tension* is applied to the muscle fiber and its contractile proteins. The tension required seems to be above two-thirds of the muscle's maximal force. If you do contractions that require little tension, you won't gain much strength. Contraction time, the total number of repetitions, also seems to influence the development of strength (Smith and Rutherford 1995). Do more contractions, and you obtain better results, up to a point. The number of contractions probably depends on your level of training, nutrition, and your genetic endowment. You will receive benefits from any form of strength training, as long as you exert enough tension for a sufficient number of repetitions (or time).

Strength = Tension × Time (number of sets and repetitions)

This chapter will help you

- understand how a bout of training leads to changes in muscles,
- identify the specific changes that result from strength or endurance training,
- recognize the importance of flexibility exercises,
- understand how to minimize muscle soreness, and
- see how speed and power training improve performance.

Muscular Fitness Training

In training we often speak of the *overload* principle, which states:

- For improvements to take place, workloads have to impose a demand (overload) on the body system (above two-thirds of maximal force for strength).
- As adaptation to loading takes place, more load must be added.
- Improvements are related to the intensity (tension for strength), duration (repetitions), and frequency of training.

Overload training leads to adaptations in the muscles according to the type of training. Here again, the principle of *specificity* applies, as it did with aerobic training. The adaptation to *strength* training includes increased size due to increases in contractile proteins (actin and myosin) and tougher connective tissue. These and other adaptations allow the muscle to exert more force.

The specific adaptations to *muscular endurance* training include improved aerobic enzyme systems, larger and more numerous mitochondria (increased mitochondrial density), and more capillaries. All these changes promote oxygen delivery and utilization within the muscle fiber, thereby improving endurance (Jackson and Dickinson 1988). Fatiguing repetitions somehow stimulate the muscle fiber to become better adapted to use oxygen and aerobic enzymes for the production of energy (adenosine triphosphate [ATP]) to sustain contractions. Perform many repetitions, and you become better able to use fat as a source of energy.

Table 9.1 reviews the effects of each type of training. It shows that high-resistance training leads to the development of strength and that low-resistance repetitions lead to muscular endurance, and suggests that there are still questions regarding the effects of training that falls between strength (high resistance and low repetitions) and endurance (low resistance and high repetitions). Use the table to help identify your training goals.

Table 9.1 The Strength-Endurance Continuum

	Strength	Short-term (anaerobic) endurance	Intermediate endurance	Long-term endurance
For	Maximum force	Brief (2-3 min) persistence with heavy load	Persistence with intermediate load	Persistence with lighter load
Prescription	6-8 RM	15-25 RM	30-50 RM	Over 100 RM
	3 sets	3 sets	2 sets	1 set
Improves	Contractile protein (actin and myosin)	Some strength and anaerobic metabolism (glycolysis)	Some endurance and anaerobic metabolism	Aerobic enzymes
	ATP and CP			Mitochondria
	Connective tissue		Slight improvement in strength (for untrained)	Oxygen and fat utilization
Doesn't improve	Oxygen intake	Oxygen intake		Strength
	Endurance			

RM = repetitions maximum
ATP = adenosine triphosphate
CP = creatine phosphate

The Training Stimulus

Just how the strength or endurance training stimuli bring about the appropriate changes is not entirely known. But from what is known about how cells work, it is likely that the training stimulus signals the nucleus to make messenger RNA (mRNA). This messenger is shaped by the DNA and sent into the muscle fiber to order the production of specific proteins (contractile protein for strength training, aerobic enzyme protein for endurance training). Structures in the muscle fiber called *ribosomes* receive the message and begin to produce the protein needed to adapt to the training stimulus. Another RNA (transfer RNA, or tRNA) is used to gather up the *amino acids* needed to construct the desired protein, transport them to the ribosome, and place them in the growing chain of amino acids that become a specific protein. Because RNA is formed by DNA, the training stimulus must somehow influence the nucleii (one muscle fiber has many). We don't know if the nucleii are signaled by tension, metabolic activity, or hormones; therefore we are unable to trick the muscle into getting stronger or building endurance without training. So you'll have to pursue the prescriptions in chapter 10 to improve your muscular strength or endurance.

Strength Training

Strength contributes to performance in work and sport, and strength training puts stresses on bones, which leads to stronger bones and a lower risk of osteoporosis. Strength training can also be used to tone muscles as well as improve your appearance and, within hereditary limits, your shape. In addition, strength training will certainly help you lead an active and vigorous life, well beyond retirement years. How does this simple mode of exercise get such remarkable results?

Strength training, also called resistance training or weight training, involves high resistance and low repetitions and leads to the following adaptations:

- Increased contractile protein (actin and myosin)
- Tougher connective tissue
- Reduced inhibitions
- Contractile efficiency
- Possible increase in number of muscle fibers

Contractile Protein

Strength training adds to the portion of the muscle that generates tension, the contractile proteins.

Years ago, Gordon (1967) compared the effects of strength and endurance training on muscle proteins. The results have since been corroborated in labs throughout the world. Strength training adds to the portion of the muscle that generates tension, the contractile proteins. Endurance training, on the other hand, enhances the energy supply system, the aerobic enzymes (all enzymes are constructed of proteins). But the most surprising outcome of his study was the observation that strength training brought about a decline in endurance enzymes, and that endurance training led to a decline in contractile protein. Thus if you train for only strength or endurance, you could lose a bit of the other. This aspect of specificity shouldn't be so surprising—the size and strength of thigh muscles increase during weight training but decline somewhat when you return to distance running.

Connective Tissue

Connective tissue and tendons grow in size and toughness when they are placed under tension. This increased toughness in tendons may help quiet the inhibitory influence of the muscle receptor known as the tendon organ, a receptor sensitive to stretching. The increase in thickness of connective tissue contributes some to the growth, or hypertrophy, of the muscle.

Nervous System

Some of the effects of strength training occur in the nervous system. With experience we seem to have fewer inhibitions, both in the central nervous system and from muscle receptors. Practice (repetition) allows us to be more efficient, more skilled in the application of force. Thus practice alone accounts for some of the improvements in the early stages of training. This may explain why involuntary contractions brought on by an electrical stimulator do not equal the results obtained with voluntary contractions. Involuntary contractions may elicit changes in the muscle, but they don't teach the nervous system how to contract (Massey et al. 1965).

Muscle Fibers

The ability to look at samples of human muscle before and after training has led to some fascinating questions. Can strength training lead to the formation of additional muscle fibers?

New Fibers?

For years we believed that the number of muscle fibers was set at birth and was not subject to change. Van Linge (1962) transplanted the tendon of a small rat muscle into a position where it would have to assume a tremendous workload. After a period of heavy training, he studied the rat muscle and found that the transplanted muscle had doubled its weight and tripled its strength. Furthermore, the heavy workload stimulated the development of new muscle fibers. Recent research indicates a role for satellite cells in muscle hypertrophy. They seem to aid regeneration of injured cells and may contribute to the formation of new fibers (Barton-Davis, Shoturma, and Sweeney 1999).

Studies on human muscle suggest that we may be able to increase the number of muscle fibers when overloaded fibers split to form new fibers. However, this finding is still the subject of scientific debate. And I would never suggest that you will form new fibers as the result of ordinary strength training. But for those athletes who spend hours each day lifting weights and also use hormones (anabolic steroids, growth hormone) to promote extra growth, increased fibers may be possible (note, however, that anabolic steroids have been found to lower HDL cholesterol and increase the risk of heart disease).

The available evidence does suggest some differences between the high-resistance/low-volume training of power lifters and the medium-resistance/high-volume training of bodybuilders. The high-resistance training seems to increase the size (hypertrophy) of fast-twitch fibers, whereas the medium-resistance/high-volume training causes selective hypertrophy of slow-twitch fibers (Tesch, Thorsson, and Kaiser 1984). Here again the response seems to be specific to the type of training.

Muscular Endurance Training

Endurance training, which involves low resistance and high repetitions, leads to the following adaptations:

- Increased aerobic enzymes
- Increased mitochondrial density
- Increased capillaries
- More efficient contractions
- Possible changes in fiber type (e.g., fast-twitch to slow-twitch)

I've already mentioned the effects of endurance training on aerobic enzymes, particularly those involved in fat metabolism; on mitochondria; and on capillaries. More efficient aerobic pathways are able to provide more energy from fat, thereby conserving muscle glycogen as well as blood glucose, which is the preferred fuel of the brain and nervous system. As a result, muscles that once fatigued in minutes become able to endure for hours. Some of the effects of endurance training take place in the nervous system. Skilled, more efficient movements conserve energy, thereby contributing to endurance. But the most documented effects of muscular endurance training seem to focus on the muscle fibers.

Fiber Type Transformation

Evidence suggests that the aerobic enzyme improvements noted in endurance training may be an early stage in the eventual transformation of fast-twitch to slow-twitch muscle fibers. Pette (1984) has reported metabolic (enzyme) and then structural changes in muscle following prolonged endurance training (electrical stimulation). Studies of rat and rabbit muscle show that fast fibers first take on improved oxidative capabilities and eventually assume the contractile properties of slow-twitch fibers. We do not yet know if these fiber type changes occur in humans.

We do know that successful distance runners have as high as 80 percent slow-twitch fibers. Is that due to fiber type transformation or to heredity? At present it appears that endurance training can improve the aerobic or oxidative capabilities of all fibers, and that fast-twitch fibers become more able to utilize oxygen. These studies demonstrate that muscle is extremely adaptable and can adjust to the demands imposed on it.

Short Versus Long Muscles

Did you ever hear that running gives you short muscles, whereas swimming gives you long ones? The truth is that the length of a muscle is fixed by its bony attachments. Running on the toes can develop the size of the calf muscle, but it isn't likely to shorten the muscle itself. Similarly, the long muscle belly seen in the calf of the swimmer could be a product of specific swim training, but it is also possible that the difference existed before training and had something to do with the athlete's success in the sport.

Methods of Training

What is the best way to train for strength or endurance: static, dynamic, or isokinetic methods? The answer depends on what you are training to accomplish, the goal of your training. If you just want to get stronger, almost any method will work. If you want to gain strength to improve performance in work or sport, your training should be specific to your goal. We conducted a study in which college women trained with weights (isotonic), isokinetic devices, or calisthenics. The isotonic group did best on lifting tests, and the calisthenics group scored best on calisthenics tests. The isokinetic training group, which gained strength on the isokinetic devices, came in third on the other two tests. This study showed how important it is to train in the manner in which the strength will eventually be used (Sharkey et al. 1978).

Static (Isometric) Training

Static contractions were the rage during the early 1960s. Professional athletes were using the technique that promised dramatic results in just six seconds a day (most unproven techniques resort to the use of celebrity claims to try to fool unsuspecting consumers). Based on an early study conducted in Germany (Hettinger and Müller 1953), the technique was popular until studies finally compared isometrics with traditional weightlifting, and static contractions came in a distant second. Isometric contractions don't provide a sense of accomplishment through lifting something, they elevate blood pressure, and they are seldom specific to the training goal. Isometrics do have some uses: in rehabilitation, when that is all that can be done; for work at the sticking point of a lift; and in activities where static strength or endurance is required (e.g., archery). More recently, isometric contractions have been used in conjunction with weightlifting to produce better results. The weight is lifted and then held against an immovable object for several counts in a technique known as functional isometrics.

Dynamic (Isotonic) Training

Isotonic contractions (weightlifting) gained popularity when DeLorme and Watkins (1951) outlined a formula for success. Simply stated, the formula called for high-resistance/low-repetition exercise. Variations of that formula are still used to develop dynamic strength. Because the resistance is high only at one point of the lift (usually the start), there has been some question about the value of the technique. Isotonic programs compare well with isokinetic training, especially when participants are tested on isotonic tests. Free weights and weight machines are readily available in most health clubs. And weightlifting with free weights remains the method of choice for most serious athletes and bodybuilders. Though fitness buffs usually lift three days a week, serious athletes increase the strength training stimulus by doing five or more sets of each exercise and by training five or six days a week.

Isokinetic Training

Isokinetic exercises combine the best features of isometric (near maximal force) and isotonic (full range of motion) training. With the appropriate device it is possible to overload the muscles with a near maximal contraction throughout the range of motion, and to control the speed of contraction. Theoretically, this method should lead to strength throughout the range of motion. The problem, if there is one, seems to be the lack of specific devices for many sports skills (see figure 9.1). But as more devices are developed for specific sports, isokinetic training may become even more popular.

Which Method Is Best?

There is no best method for strength or endurance training. Free weights are inexpensive and versatile but require more supervision for safety and to prevent theft. Weight machines are convenient and require less supervision. Isokinetic devices are effective but limited in application. Variable and accommodating resistance devices adjust the resistance to the available force. Popular in health clubs, they are useful for fitness and sport and have one special advantage: Unlike weightlifting, isokinetic training doesn't cause muscle soreness. Thus it can be done in conjunction with other activities without adversely affecting performance.

A note of caution before we go on: Be sure the training program you adopt is appropriate to your level of fitness and ability. What is best for beginners doesn't work for athletes, and vice versa. In psychology many theories are based on

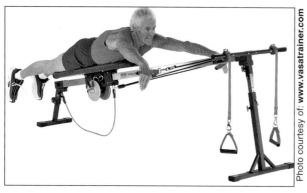

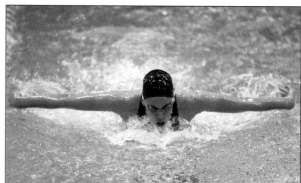

Photo courtesy of: www.vasatrainer.com

Figure 9.1 *(a)* The swim bench provides a sport-specific way to train. *(b)* A swimmer training.

research conducted on college freshmen and rats. In exercise physiology, numerous studies have been conducted on "gym rats," college students enrolled in activity classes. When various forms of strength training are compared on gym rats, they all seem to yield similar results; in other words, follow the prescription and anything works—with beginners. But that doesn't predict how the method will work on athletes or others with higher levels of strength. And it doesn't prove that the increased strength will improve performance. We know how to improve strength. Now we need to find out how much is needed to improve performance, and how best to train to get results (chapter 10).

Flexibility

To consider the effect of training on range of motion, first we must consider the limits of flexibility. Muscles are covered with tough connective tissue, and this tissue is a major restriction to the range of motion, as are the joint capsule and tendons. Thus training must concentrate on altering these limits. Flexibility decreases with age and inactivity. Some injuries may be more likely as flexibility decreases, and low back problems are associated with poor flexibility (back, hamstrings) and weak abdominal muscles. On the other hand, enhanced flexibility may improve performance in some sports, especially those with obvious flexibility components (gymnastics, diving, wrestling).

Increased muscle and joint temperatures increase flexibility, as do specific stretching exercises. Stretching gradually leads to minor distensions in connective tissue, and the summation of these small changes can be a dramatically improved range of motion.

Years ago, flexibility exercises conjured up images of vigorous bobbing and jerking movements, but times have changed. Today we engage in static stretching or, at most, light bobbing movements. The reason for the change is the stretch reflex. A rapid stretch invokes a stretch reflex, and the reflex calls forth a vigorous contraction of the muscle. Because a vigorous contraction is the opposite of what we are seeking, we must avoid this explosive stretching and learn the gentle art and science of static stretching.

Static Stretching

Static stretching involves slow movements to reach a point of stretch, holding the position (5 to 10 seconds), and relaxing. The stretch may be repeated, and very light bobbing may be employed. A variation of the static stretch is the contract/relax technique. Do a static stretch, relax, then contract the muscle for a few seconds. Then repeat the static stretch. When performed on muscles like those in the calf, the technique seems to help the muscle relax so you can better stretch the tendon. These methods are at least as effective as dynamic stretching, and they provide other advantages such as low risk of injury and reduction of tightness and lingering muscle soreness.

Warm up a bit with light exercise or calisthenics, then do your stretching. Finish the warm-up with more vigorous effort or, if you prefer, begin your run or other exercise at a slow pace. Never substitute skill rehearsal, such as tennis strokes, for stretching. Do your warm-up and stretching before you begin to compete. When flexibility training is done correctly, the results are quite persistent. Your improved range of motion should remain for at least eight weeks. But once you have learned to enjoy stretching, you may get hooked on its subtle sensations and move on to advanced forms such as yoga. If not, just remember to do the stretches you need to minimize soreness, to reduce the risk of injury, and to avoid low back problems (see figure 9.2).

Muscle Soreness

The muscle soreness that becomes evident 24 hours after you overdo training (delayed-onset muscle soreness, or DOMS) may be due to slight tears in connective tissue, to uncontrolled contractions or spasms of individual muscle fibers, to muscle fiber damage, or to the lingering effects of metabolic by-products. We are reasonably certain that soreness is not due to leftover lactic acid. That by-product is eliminated within an hour of the cessation of effort. We do know that certain types of exercise (but not isokinetic) lead to soreness that often persists for days and can make subsequent activity less enjoyable. Komi and Buskirk (1972) compared two types of strength training: concentric (as in ordinary flexion) and eccentric (the muscle is under high tension as it lowers an overload). Subjects in the eccentric group, the group that lowered the weight, complained of muscle soreness, whereas the other group did not. So if you begin a weightlifting program and plan to lower the weights, be prepared for some soreness.

You can diminish soreness by beginning with light weights and progressing gradually. Avoid maximal lifting, all-out running, or ballistic movements such as hard throwing or serving at the start of the season. Be patient. Experience shows that we are seldom patient enough; therefore, we need a way to reduce soreness. Stretching has been shown to reduce muscle discomfort (deVries 1986), so stretch before and after exercise and whenever you feel tight or sore. If your legs are stiff and sore during a long flight, go to the rear of the plane and stretch. If other passengers see you trying to push down the wall of the galley, don't be embarrassed. Fitness enthusiasts will understand that you are experiencing the pleasure and relief of a good static stretch.

Muscle soreness is correlated with submicroscopic muscle damage, accumulation of fluid (edema), and diminished strength that may persist for up to two weeks. The damage may be to older or otherwise susceptible muscle fibers. Recovery is faster and soreness is diminished after successive bouts of exercise. Leakage of the muscle enzyme creatine kinase (CK) suggests membrane damage. Because the soreness peaks one to two days after the effort, and the enzyme levels peak two to three days later, the actual cause of the muscle soreness is still unclear (Newham 1988). Fortunately DOMS occurs only during the start-up phase, and

Muscle soreness is correlated with submicroscopic muscle damage, accumulation of fluid (edema), and diminished strength that may persist for up to two weeks.

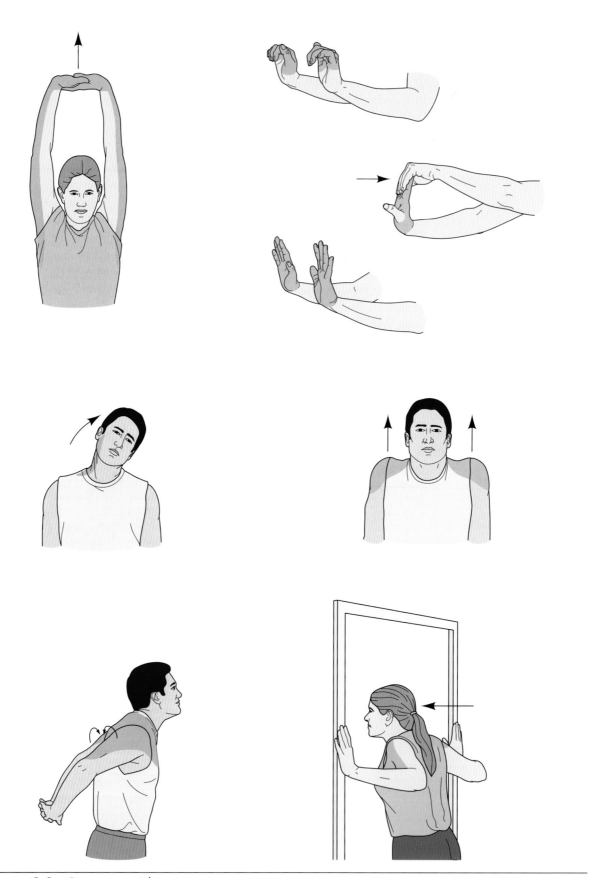

Figure 9.2 Common stretching exercises.

Adapted from Stretching, Inc.

10

Improving Your Muscular Fitness

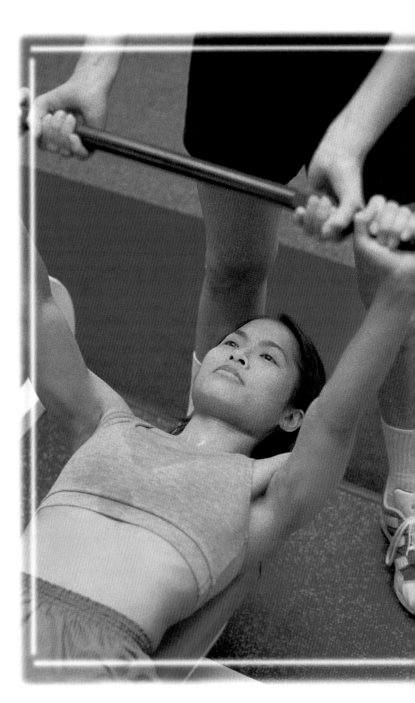

"The two kinds of people on earth . . . are the people who lift and the people who lean."

Ella Wheeler Wilcox

By now you have some idea of the benefits and applications of muscular fitness. First and foremost are the health benefits; all of us need to do flexibility and abdominal exercises to prevent low back problems. Try to maintain a regular schedule. If you don't, you are likely to become one of the millions of Americans whose days are diminished by this preventable problem. Those at risk for osteoporosis should plan a prevention program that consists of moderate weightlifting along with weight-bearing aerobic activity. And middle-aged individuals must understand how muscular fitness contributes to muscle mass, mobility, and the quality of life after retirement, and realize that they should begin long before they retire and continue the rest of their days.

Of course, there are many other reasons to improve muscular fitness; many people become involved to correct posture or perceived deficiencies of figure or physique (e.g., to look good at the beach). Body shaping and bodybuilding motivate many participants. To help decide on a program, you may also want to evaluate your current level of muscular fitness. If you are dissatisfied, if there is room for improvement, or if you want to enhance performance in work or sport, use the prescriptions, select your mode of exercise, and get going. You'll be happy to learn that muscular fitness doesn't have to take a lot of time. Unless you are seeking high levels of strength or endurance, you should be able to achieve health and other goals with two to three weekly sessions of 30 minutes each. And you can maintain muscular fitness with one or two sessions per week.

This chapter will help you

- develop training prescriptions for muscular strength, endurance, speed, and power;
- take precautions and follow guidelines to make training safe and effective; and
- adopt a program to improve or maintain low back fitness.

Warm-Up

Warm-up is as important for you as it is for your car. During winter months you can't just jump into the old pickup and expect instant performance; you start the engine and wait a few seconds while the oil pressure rises. Then you drive slowly to avoid overloading the engine until it heats up. In the case of the body, muscle is the engine, and increased muscle temperature improves enzyme activity and combustion. By slowly increasing heart rate, respiration, and muscle temperature, you avoid wasteful and uncomfortable anaerobic metabolism early in the workout. And by slowly stretching and warming the muscles, you greatly reduce the risk of injury (use the exercises in chapter 9). A five-minute warm-up before and a cool-down after exercise will enhance your enjoyment of the experience and increase the likelihood that you will be able to participate tomorrow, without discomfort. And remember, muscular fitness is only part of total fitness; no program is complete without a well-planned aerobic fitness regimen.

Prescriptions for Muscular Strength

Research has identified safe, proven prescriptions for each component of muscular fitness. You may fulfill the prescription with calisthenics, weights, or weight machines. You'll get results with hydraulic devices, accommodating or variable resistance equipment, or old-fashioned free weights. The key is to place the muscle under tension (at least two-thirds of maximal strength) for a sufficient time (repetitions and sets). How you intend to use the strength will dictate how you should train. Training is specific in terms of angle, range of motion, and even velocity of contractions. Train the muscles and movements you are anxious to improve. In designing your program, consider the factors described in the following sections.

Repetitions

We've known how to prescribe strength training since the early 50s, when DeLorme and Watkins (1951) published their analysis of progressive resistance exercise. This report and more recent studies have confirmed the need to use a resistan ce that can be lifted up to 10 times (repetitions maximum, or RM); when more repetitions are possible, the load must be increased (hence the term progressive resistance). A comprehensive review of the literature leads to the conclusion that there is no one optimal number of repetitions. Anything between 2 and 10 RM yields success, as long as each set is in fact the maximal number of repetitions possible (Fleck and Kraemer 1997). Of course, it is safer to work at the higher end of that range, so 6 to 10 repetitions are usually prescribed for all but the most serious lifters.

Sets

Although a study with adult recreational lifters suggests that a single set provides an adequate training stimulus (Hass et al. 2000), other studies show that three sets of up to 10 RM yield as much as 50 percent more (Kramer et al. 1997). Later in this chapter I'll point out how more sets are used in advanced weight training. A prudent approach is to begin with one set of each exercise, then progress to two and then three sets as strength develops.

Frequency

One of the early studies to compare different training frequencies (Barham 1960) found that three- or five-day-per-week formats were superior to two per week; but the three- and five-day programs were not significantly different from each other. In their 1997 review, Fleck and Kraemer concluded that the majority of research indicates that three training sessions per muscle group per week is the minimum frequency which causes *maximum* gains in strength. Apparently, it takes untrained individuals 48 hours to recover from a training bout and to adapt to the training stimulus.

The basic prescription for strength is:

- Three sets of 6 to 10 RM
- Three times per week (every other day)

In practice many lifters prefer to vary the program by changing the number of repetitions per set. Some begin at 10 RM, then go to 8 and end at 6; others prefer to begin low and go up (e.g., 6, 8, and 10 RM). For safety's sake I recommend you begin with more reps and less weight and avoid high weights (low RM). Just remember to increase the resistance when you are able to do more than 10 reps in all three sets. Keep in mind that most of the studies that led to these conclusions were done on "gym rats," previously untrained (novice) students enrolled in college physical education classes. The prescription for advanced lifting is more demanding.

Guidelines

If you engage in calisthenics, weight training, or isokinetics, keep the following points in mind:

- Ease into the program with lighter weights and fewer sets.
- Avoid holding your breath during a lift. This can cause a marked increase in blood pressure and the work of the heart. It also restricts the return of blood to the heart and the flow of blood in the coronary arteries that serve the heart muscle (just when your heart needs more oxygen, it gets less—a dangerous situation, especially for older, untrained individuals). Breath holding can also increase intra-abdominal pressure and cause a hernia.
- Exhale during the lift and inhale as you lower the weight.
- Always work with a companion or spotter when using free weights.
- Alternate muscle groups during a session; don't do several arm exercises in a row. Allow recovery time between sets of the same exercise.

Also, you should take the following measures.

- Keep records of your progress. Test for maximum strength every few weeks (see figure 10.1 for a log to keep track of progress). Also record body weight and fat, and some dimensions (chest, waist, biceps, etc.).
- Vary the program. Experienced athletes use a process called cycling (or periodization) that usually includes four cycles of four weeks each or longer. For example, Fleck and Kraemer (1997) suggest this program for athletes in high-strength sports. Simply follow each of the four-week cycles:

  1. 10 to 20 reps, low resistance—for hypertrophy
  2. 2 to 6 reps, medium resistance—for strength
  3. 2 to 3 reps, high resistance—for added strength
  4. 1 to 3 reps, very high resistance—peaking phase

Each cycle can be as short as four weeks or as long as eight. Because progress begins to plateau after two months, I prefer to change my program every eight weeks. Another approach is to change exercises every four to eight weeks, or when you plateau or get bored. In chapter 16 I will show you how you can use cycling or periodization in training for performance in sport.

Muscular Fitness Log

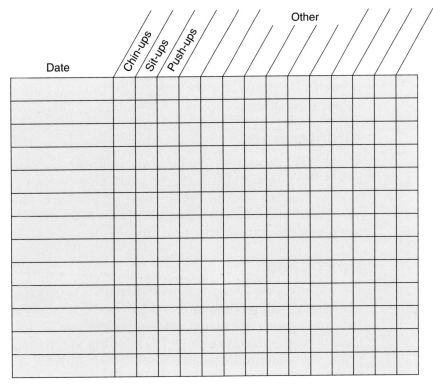

Figure 10.1 Muscular fitness log.

Progress

Although strength doesn't increase rapidly, you can expect the following:

- Your rate of increase will range from 1 to 3 percent per week, with previously untrained individuals increasing at a faster rate. With hard training, some people may temporarily achieve a rate of 4 to 5 percent per week.

- The rate of improvement will decrease or plateau as you approach your potential maximal strength.

- The rate of improvement may be slowed if you combine strength training with strenuous aerobic training.

- Improvements will take place only in the muscle groups you train.
- Gains will be minimized if you fail to maintain adequate protein and energy in your diet. Increase protein intake if you are on a weight-loss diet.

A previously sedentary individual on an adequate diet can expect to increase strength 50 percent or more in six months. Hard training could lead to similar gains in less time.

Maintenance

You can maintain strength with lower volume and frequency of training, as long as intensity (resistance) remains high. One session per week will maintain strength for six weeks or more; two sessions will ensure maintenance for a prolonged period, depending on the level of strength you achieved before beginning the maintenance program.

Detraining

Studies on older individuals show that strength declines very slowly in those muscle groups that are used regularly.

With normal activity, newly gained strength is largely retained for up to six weeks after the cessation of training, and half of the strength you gain will be retained for up to one year. When you resume training, you'll return to previous levels with less effort, perhaps because of the learning that took place in earlier training. Studies on older individuals show that strength declines very slowly in those muscle groups that are used regularly. Thus an investment in strength could pay dividends later in life. Of course, I would recommend that you set aside at least 8 to 12 weeks each year to maintain or improve strength, and to continue a maintenance program thereafter. Find a season that suits your schedule and follow a program. As the years pass, you'll be glad you did.

Advanced Strength Training

Experienced lifters train six days per week. When they engage in bodybuilding, they do many sets and repetitions. Training for superior strength calls for numerous sets (more than 10) with few repetitions and very heavy loads. Some of these athletes have been known to take protein supplements or even drugs to enhance their progress. Research supports an increase of *dietary* protein when the athlete is on a weight-loss (energy-deficient) diet (Butterfield 1987).

Anabolic Steroids

The use of steroid drugs to improve performance has become commonplace in the world of sports, especially bodybuilding, football, and professional wrestling. Though the effects of steroids on strength have been supported by some research, their use is dangerous and unhealthy. Anabolic steroids affect glandular function, damage the liver, and lead to early heart disease via an alarming drop in HDL cholesterol. Furthermore, they have been associated with testicular atrophy, psychological rage, and other problems. Don't depend on steroids, growth hormone, or any other drug for strength or performance.

Advanced strength training guidelines include the following:

- Work up to five or six sets.
- Utilize a split program: upper body on Monday, Wednesday, and Friday; trunk and legs on Tuesday, Thursday, and Saturday.
- Consume adequate energy and protein (1.6 grams per kilogram of body weight), avoid rapid weight loss, and get ample rest.
- Cut back on endurance training unless you are very fit (best results may occur when serious strength training is conducted separately) (Hickson 1980).
- Use training cycles; change your program every four to eight weeks or when progress begins to plateau.

Strength may be related to performance in your work or sport. If so, by all means train to improve your strength. However, don't assume (as many have) that if some is good, more is better. In most activities, performance improves with strength, but only to a point. Thereafter, you may be wasting your time or diminishing performance with excessive attention to strength. The trick is to know how much is enough. When strength is optimal for the sport, move on to other important phases of training. Just be sure to maintain the necessary strength with one or two sessions each week.

How Much Is Enough?

How much strength is sufficient? The answer differs according to the sport. For an endurance sport such as swimming or cross-country skiing, strength is adequate when the force needed in a single contraction (e.g., the arm pull in swimming) is below 40 percent of your maximal for that movement. If you exert 20 pounds of force in the average arm pull, you need approximately 50 pounds of force (2.5 times 20 pounds) in a single maximal pull. More strength will not contribute to performance; if the arm pulls through too quickly, you'll go slower, not faster. So if strength is adequate, move on to endurance training. For daylong work, strength is adequate when the force needed is at or below 20 percent of your maximal. If a loaded shovel weighs 10 pounds, you'll need 50 pounds of force (5 times 10) (I'll say more about strength and performance in chapters 15 and 16).

Prescriptions for Muscular Endurance

I've pointed out how strength and endurance are different and why endurance may be more important than a high level of strength, presuming that you have adequate strength. The main difference between training for strength and training for endurance is the level of tension in the muscle and, consequently, the resistance used and number of repetitions possible. Lighter weights (less than 66 percent of maximum strength) don't provide much stimulus for strength development, but if you do enough repetitions, you will develop muscular endurance.

Years ago it was believed that training with fewer than 10 RM developed strength, whereas training with more than 10 RM developed endurance. I wondered if the body really made such fine distinctions. Recent studies have added to our knowledge of strength and endurance and the territory that lies between. Studies in our lab (Washburn et al. 1982) and others (Anderson and Kearney 1982) show that 15 to 25 RM will still develop some strength (1 percent per week versus 2 to 3 percent with 6 to 10 RM for strength training), along with short-term or anaerobic endurance. Table 10.1 describes the strength-endurance continuum and includes a summary of the effects of various numbers of repetitions and what they are likely to develop. As the number of repetitions increases, less strength and more endurance is developed.

Table 10.1   The Strength-Endurance Continuum

	Strength	Short-term (anaerobic) endurance	Intermediate endurance	Long-term endurance
Train with	High resistance	Medium resistance		Low resistance
	Low repetitions	Medium repetitions		High repetitions
Training effect	More contractile proteins (actin and myosin)		?	Aerobic enzymes and mitochondria
	Increased short-term energy (ATP and CP)			Improved oxygen intake and fat utilization
	Stronger connective tissue			Increased capillaries
	Reduced inhibitions			

ATP = adenosine triphosphate
CP = creatine phosphate

The number of repetitions you need depends on several factors. What are you training for? Is it for short-term (anaerobic) or for long-term endurance? Training should be specific to the way in which it will be used. Emphasize speed when necessary. Do many repetitions when long-term endurance with less resistance is needed. When the activity involves moderate resistance, lift heavier weights and do fewer repetitions. For short (under two minutes) and intense activities, train with 15 to 25 RM to get short-term or anaerobic endurance. If your goals are vague and time is short, use fewer repetitions. A friend once worked up to 400 sit-ups daily, then quit because he became bored. (Incidentally, he didn't get rid of his tummy fat until diet and aerobic exercise led to general weight loss.)

Follow the appropriate endurance prescription and observe the precautions mentioned for strength training. However, because the loads are lighter, muscle endurance training is safer than strength training, and it is probably more related to the everyday activities of the average adult.

Progress

Muscle endurance is very trainable. Though it is difficult to go from two to four chin-ups (that takes strength), it is easy to improve from 20 to 40 push-ups (that

Most adult activities are enhanced when endurance is improved.

takes endurance). When you have sufficient strength for the task, gains in endurance come with relative ease. Subjects in the Washburn study improved 10 percent per week in short-term endurance when they trained with 15 to 25 RM. On a laboratory endurance test, the short-term (anaerobic) endurance training was more effective than strength training, improving short-term endurance 70 percent versus 50 percent for strength training. Most adult activities are enhanced when endurance is improved. Tennis and skiing require hours of practice, and good practice requires endurance. The fatigued tennis student usually practices a sloppy version of the skill, and a fatigued skier carries a higher risk of injury.

Of course, your ultimate progress will be dictated by your genetic endowment and your devotion to training. If you have a high percentage of slow-twitch muscle fibers, your potential for muscular endurance is excellent. If you do not, don't despair; training will improve the endurance capabilities of all fiber types. Though you may not be a world-class endurance athlete, you will come closer to your potential.

Diet and Endurance

The best endurance performances happen when muscle fibers are well supplied with muscle glycogen. And glycogen levels are highest when you follow a high-carbohydrate diet. Scandinavian studies have shown that muscle glycogen stores can be depleted in a full day of alpine skiing. If you dine on steak and salad after skiing, your muscles will not be ready to perform the following day. Do all you can to replace muscle glycogen, and you will be able to ski all day and still have energy for après-ski. More important, you will be less likely to fatigue, fall, and get injured. Begin carbohydrate replacement immediately after activity and continue with a high-carbohydrate diet (see the performance diet in chapter 11).

Circuit Weight Training

Circuit weight training (CWT) involves a series of weight training exercises designed to promote strength and muscular endurance. The CWT circuit, with short rest intervals between sets, is intended to raise energy expenditure and heart rate, and—according to some fitness practitioners—to improve aerobic fitness. Though this popular technique will improve strength and muscular endurance, its effect on aerobic fitness is slight (3 to 5 percent). A set of 10 repetitions of an exercise such as a forearm curl is not sufficient to overload the oxidative system of the muscle. So its effect on aerobic fitness is far less than the 20 to 25 percent improvement derived from sustained large-muscle activity such as cycling or running. Aerobic fitness improvements are increased when you jog between sets.

However, CWT is an effective way to achieve muscular fitness goals, but whether the rest interval between sets is short (20 seconds) or long (60 seconds), the effect on energy expenditure or aerobic fitness is modest at best (Haltom et al. 1999). My advice? Do CWT if you like, but if you want the most from muscular and aerobic fitness training, do each individually.

Prescriptions for Speed and Power

As with other types of training, the key to speed and power training is specificity. Try to pattern the training after the intended use. To throw a baseball faster, train with a weighted ball or simulate the motion with pulley weights or an isokinetic device. To improve jumping ability, do half squats with weights, jump while wearing a weighted vest, or use an isokinetic jumping device. When in doubt, be specific. Here are some ideas on speed and power training.

- **Speed (velocity):** Do high-speed contractions with low resistance. Sprinters have gained speed by running downhill, running against resistance, and assisted running (being towed). For more on speed training consult a good book on the subject (e.g., Dintiman and Ward 1988).

- **Power (force × velocity):** Do three sets of 15 to 25 high-speed contractions with 30 to 60 percent of maximal resistance. You can use accommodating resistance devices to do power training, but free weights are not well suited to this high-speed training.

Another approach, a popular technique borrowed from European coaches, is *plyometrics.* Plyometrics are explosive movements designed to improve power. Sprinters do one- and two-leg hops to gain power. High jumpers, broad jumpers, volleyball and basketball athletes, and even cross-country skiers use plyometrics in an attempt to improve performance. Proponents have said that plyometrics train the capacity for preload/elastic recoil and build strength and explosive power (Radcliffe and Farentinos 1985). Unfortunately, the limited research remains inconclusive concerning the value of plyometrics for various sports and for athletes at different levels of development. And excessive use or poor technique can lead to painful knee problems. I recommend that you try plyometrics, if only because of the effect of practice on skill and economy. But start with a modest number, on a soft surface, and quit at the first sign of discomfort in the knee. Even if you don't gain additional power, you may become more effective in the use of the power you possess (In chapter 9 I described the phenomenon called preload/elastic recoil, and told how it contributes to power and performance.) The following are a few plyometrics exercises.

■ Hops

Do one-leg hops, alternating legs with a balance step between hops. Do 10 with each leg; work up to two sets of 20.

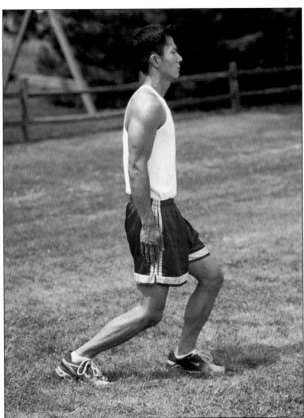

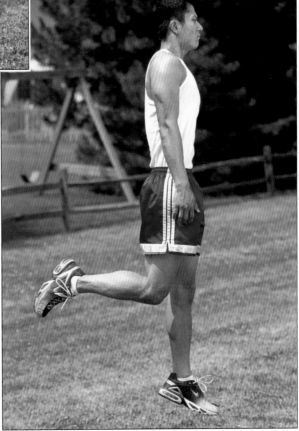

■ Two-Leg Jumps

Jump as high as possible from both legs. Do 10 to 20 explosive two-leg jumps.

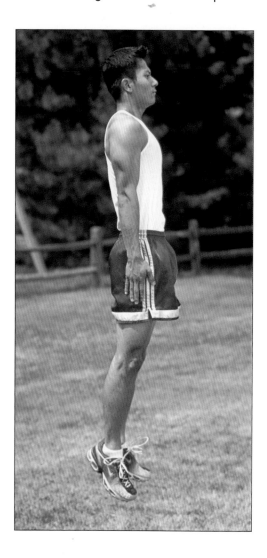

■ Squat Jumps

Stand with hands on hips, one foot a step ahead of the other. Squat (drop quickly) until your front thigh is at a 90-degree angle to the lower leg, then immediately jump as high as possible, extending the knees. Switch position of feet on the way down, land, squat, and jump again. Perform 10 to 20 repetitions.

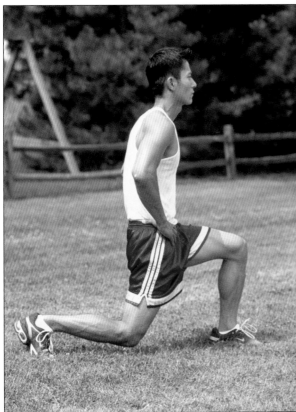

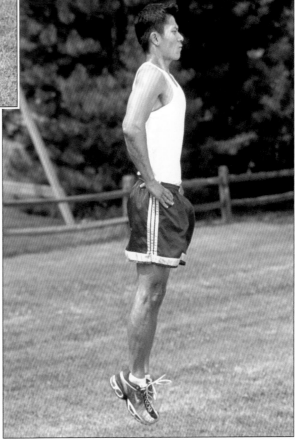

Specificity

The concept of specificity applies to muscular fitness training and testing. Training is specific in regard to angle and speed, and static tests do not reflect the effects of dynamic training (Baker, Wilson, and Carlyon 1994). High-resistance training yields greater strength gains, whereas low-resistance training produces greater gains in muscular endurance (Morrissey, Harman, and Johnson 1995). For best results, train specifically.

Calisthenics

Calisthenics include a wide range of exercises, such as push-ups, chin-ups, and sit-ups. The strength training prescription calls for high resistance and low repetitions, so you may have to add additional resistance when you are able to do more than 10 repetitions (more than 10 repetitions will build short-term endurance but not much strength). You can overload the push-up in several ways. For example, have someone place a hand on your back to increase the resistance, or put your feet on a chair to place more weight on the arms. You could also do variations, such as fingertip push-ups or power push-ups (push up and clap hands). Just remember, as the repetitions exceed 10, you are shifting toward endurance training. Calisthenics can be used to train for both. Try the following calisthenics exercises.

■ Knee Push-Up

This is a good chest and triceps exercise for beginners. With hands outside your shoulders and knees bent, push up, keeping your back straight. Do as many as possible.

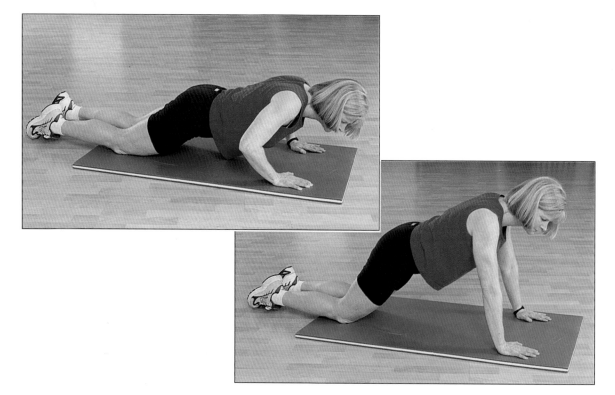

■ Push-Up

This is an intermediate exercise. With hands outside your shoulders, push up, keeping your back straight; return until your chest almost touches the floor. Do as many as possible.

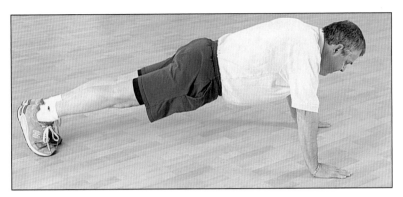

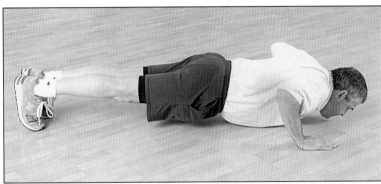

■ Chair Dips

This is an advanced exercise. Make sure the chair you use is stationary. Grasp the sides of the chair, and slide your feet forward while supporting your weight on your arms. Lower your body, and return. Do as many as possible. You can also use parallel bars if available.

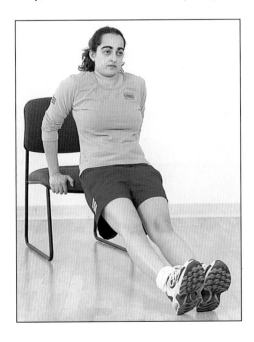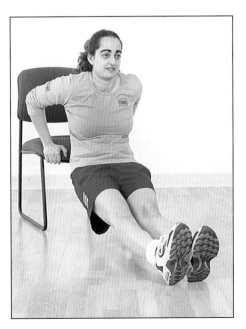

■ **Modified Chin-Up**

This is a biceps and back exercise for beginners. Stand with the bar about chest height. With an underhand grasp, hang from the bar with the body straight and feet on the ground. Pull up, and return. Do as many as possible.

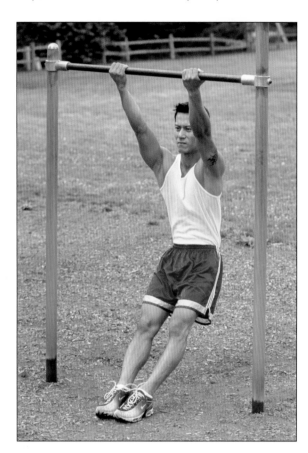

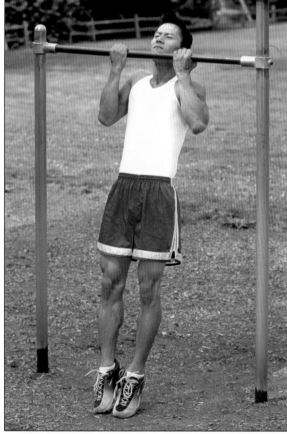

Chin-Up

This is the intermediate version of the exercise. With the underhand grasp, pull up until your chin is over the bar; return. Do as many as possible. Variations include using an overhand grip or climbing a rope.

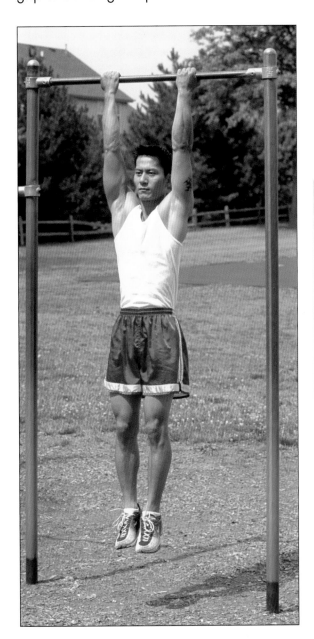

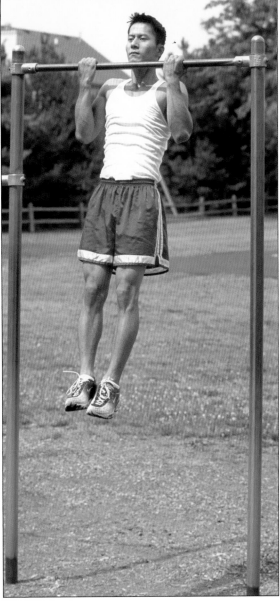

Fitness and Health

◼ Pike Chin-Up

This is an advanced exercise. Perform the chin-up from the bar with legs in a pike position.

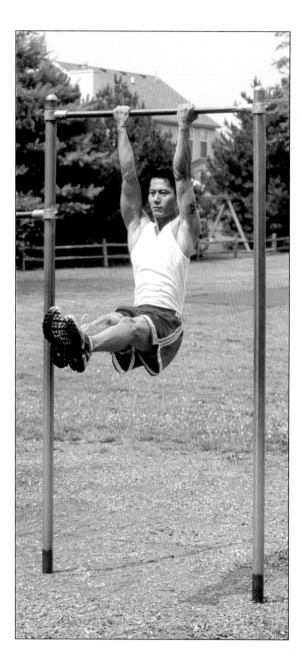

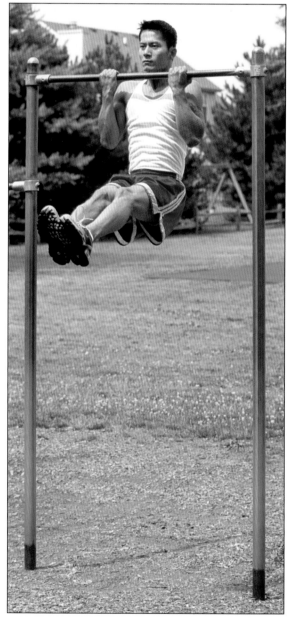

■ Sit-Up With Arms Crossed

This is a good exercise for abdominal strength and endurance. On your back with arms crossed on the chest and knees bent, curl up to a semi-sitting position, and return. Do 10 to 15 times. Variations: Do repetitions very fast; do the exercise on an inclined board; hold a weight on your chest.

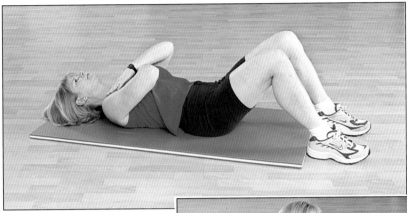

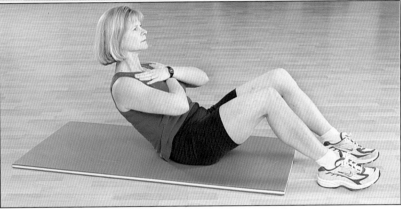

■ Hills

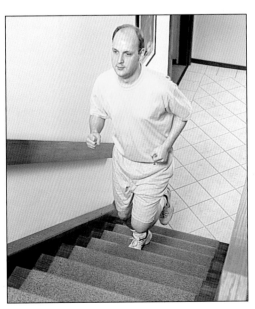

Power walk up a steep hill, stadium steps, or office stairs. Variations: Use ski poles for balance, to aid the downhill trip, or to exercise arms. Wear a weighted pack for added resistance.

■ Basket Hang

This is a more advanced exercise. Hang from the bar with an underhand grasp. Raise your legs into a "basket," and return. Do as many as possible.

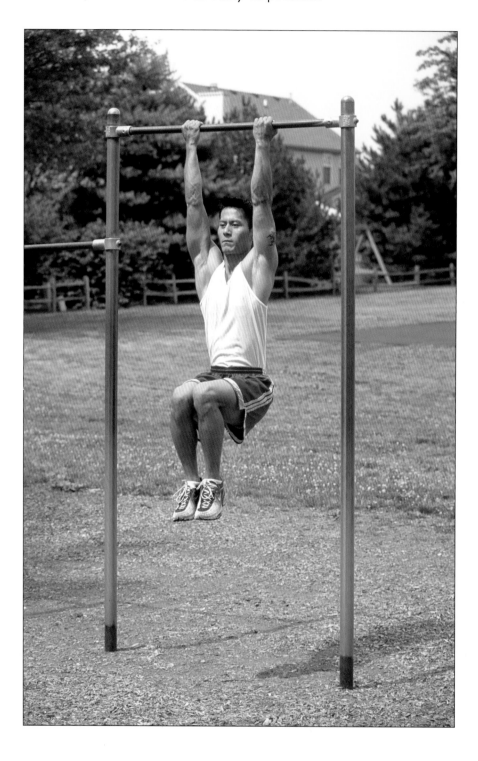

■ Leg Lifts

This is a good exercise for back strength and endurance. Lying facedown on the floor, with a partner holding your trunk down, raise your legs 5 to 10 times. Avoid hyperextension.

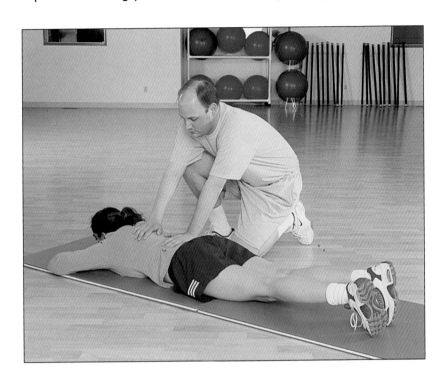

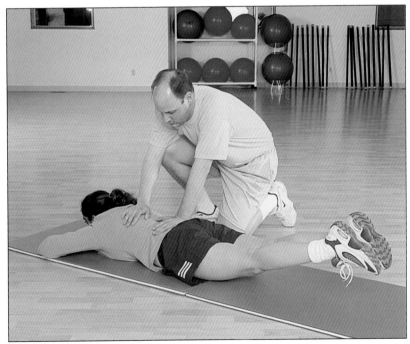

Trunk Lifts

Lying facedown on the floor with fingers laced behind your head and ankles anchored to the ground, raise your trunk 5 to 10 times. Don't overextend.

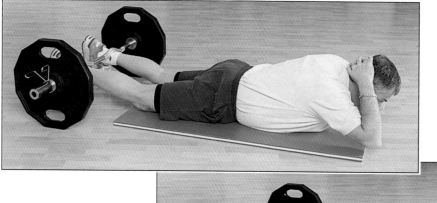

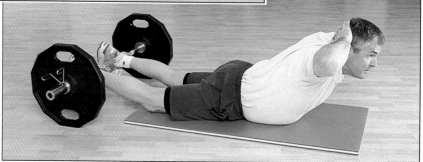

Bench Stepping

Step up and down on a bench as fast as possible for 30 seconds. Switch lead leg and repeat. Bench stepping can also be done with a loaded pack.

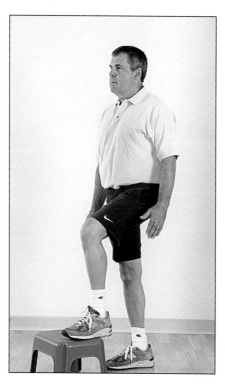

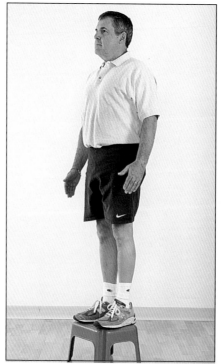

■ Half Knee Bends

This exercise is good for leg strength and endurance. With feet apart and hands on hips, squat until your thighs are parallel to the ground; return. Do as many as possible. Try a 2-inch (5-centimeter) block under the heels to aid balance. For variety, do this exercise with a weight on your back (e.g., a backpack).

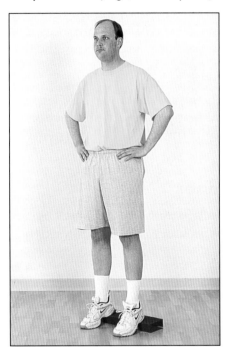 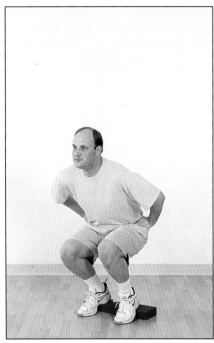

■ Heel Raises

Stand erect, hands at sides or on hips, feet close together. Raise up on your toes 20 to 40 times. Heel raises can be done with toes on a 2-inch (5-centimeter) platform; or do them with a loaded pack.

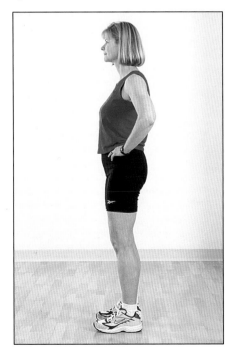 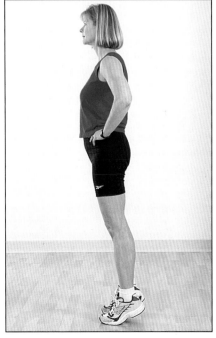

Weight Training

Weight training, sometimes called resistance training, has emerged as an essential part of the program to improve performance, fitness, and even health. Use a weight training apparatus (stack weights) or free weights (bar and weights). Though machines are expensive, they have several advantages over free weights: They are safer and more versatile, they save time, and they eliminate equipment theft. Using a machine also makes it much easier to change resistance as you move from one exercise to another. On the negative side, a machine restricts you to a set series of lifts and movements, and you don't learn to balance the load as well. But for general training, and especially for groups, the machines are probably the best bet. Try the weight training exercises that follow the descriptions of the apparatus in this section. Remember, for strength, do three sets of 6 to 10 repetitions, three times per week (every other day).

Weight Training Machines

Several companies manufacture weight training machines. Universal Gym, popular isotonic equipment, typically provides stations for the bench press and leg press, as well as the following:

- Abdomen and trunk exercises
- Military press and curls
- Lat pull-down
- Leg flexion and extension

Nautilus equipment utilizes a cam to adjust resistance throughout the lift. Most clubs have stations for triceps and chest exercises and the leg press, as well as the following:

- Biceps curl
- Bench press
- Lat pull-over and pull-down
- Leg flexion and extension
- Abdominals and trunk

Mini Gym makes a variety of variable-resistance devices specifically designed for certain sports such as basketball, volleyball, and swimming. Excellent equipment is also manufactured by Paramount, Hydra Gym, Kaiser, Polaris, and others. Sturdy home devices are now available for $1,000 to $2,500.

Free Weights

Advanced programs often utilize free weights to isolate and overload specific muscles. Use the appropriate prescription to achieve your goal (e.g., 6 to 10 repetitions maximum for strength).

■ Leg Press

Leg presses work the quadriceps. Place your feet on the pedals and grasp the handles of the seat. Press your feet forward to elevate the weight, and return. Inhale while lowering the weight and exhale while lifting it.

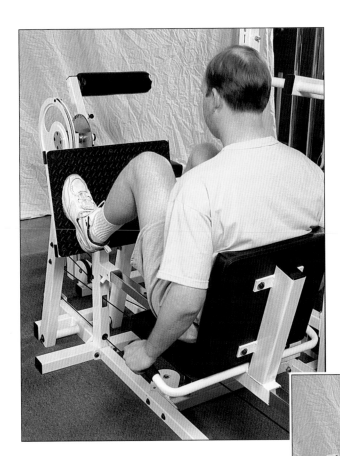

■ Leg Flexion

This exercise works the hamstrings. Lie facedown on the table with heels positioned behind the padded bar. Flex your legs to elevate the weight. Return to the starting position. Watch for leg cramps.

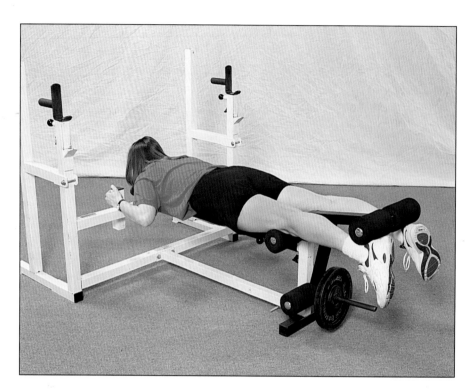

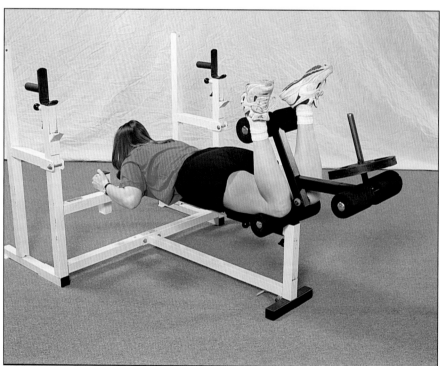

■ Leg Extension

This works the quadriceps. Sit on the bench, with your instep under the padded bar. Extend your legs to elevate the weight. Return to starting position.

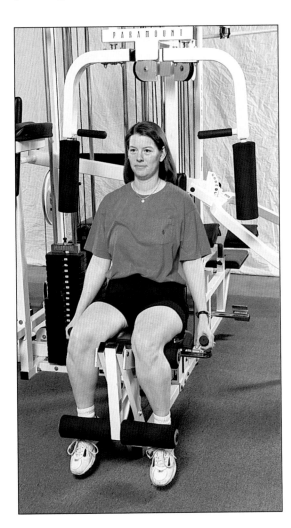 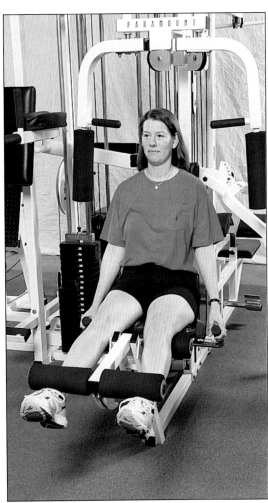

Isokinetics

Isokinetic devices, as well as variable and accommodating resistance machines, are available in health and fitness clubs, in recreation centers, in schools and colleges, and even in private homes. The good ones allow you to exert near-maximum force as the device moves through a full range of motion. You can vary the speed and resistance to suit specific training needs. Low-cost home devices can be used in a variety of ways. Least expensive of all is isokinetic exercise with a friend (counterforce). Your partner provides resistance throughout the range of motion; for example, as you attempt forearm flexion, your partner provides resistance (see the following exercises). You can do fast, medium, or slow isokinetics, depending on the goal of your training. But recent studies indicate that moderately fast training against resistance is more likely to develop strength and power.

Follow the program on an alternating-day schedule. Select the program to suit your needs, not those of the club. If you need medium or fast contractions for your sport, do them. Also, if they say to do one set, take their advice for the first eight weeks. But when your strength plateaus, as it will with one set, progress to two and then three sets. Fitness clubs like slow contractions that save wear and tear on the machines, and they advise one set not because it is the best way to train, but because it avoids long waits to use the apparatus.

■ Arm Flexion

As partner 1 tries to lift her arms, partner 2 resists the movement. Partner 2 should allow movement to progress slowly (range of motion in three seconds). Do three sets of eight repetitions.

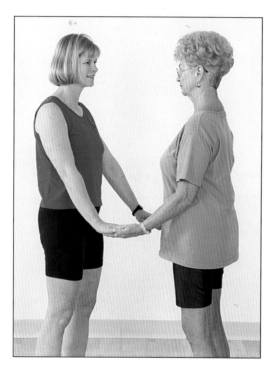

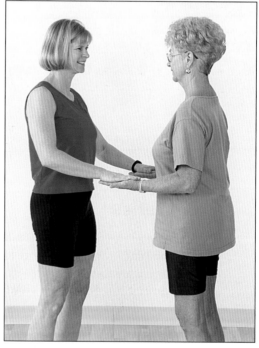

Double Knee Pull

Starting in the same position, with your arms at your sides, draw your knees to your chest and clasp your hands around your knees. Keeping your shoulders flat against the floor, pull your knees tightly against your chest, hold 10 seconds, and relax; repeat. Repeat and touch your forehead to your knees.

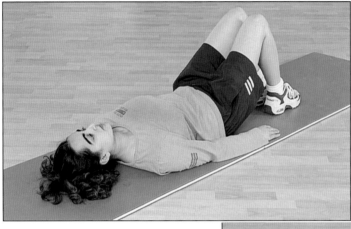

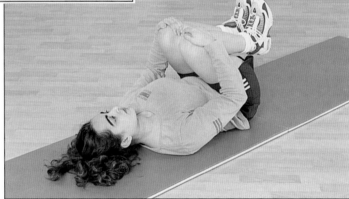

Angry Cat

Kneel and place your hands on the floor. Lower your head and contract your abdominal and buttocks muscles, arch your lower back, hold 5 seconds, and relax.

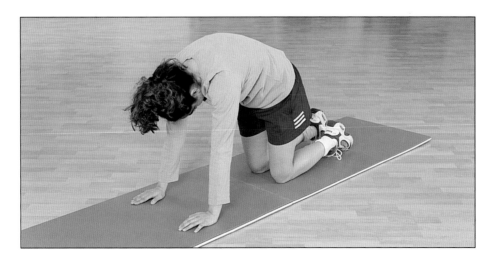

Curl-Up

Bend your knees with your feet flat on the floor; lift one leg and rest the ankle on the knee of the opposite leg. Lock your hands behind your head. Raise your head and shoulders from the floor. With chin to chest and with back rounded, curl up as far as possible, trying to touch your elbow to the opposite knee. Be sure to pull with the abdominal muscles. Lower slowly. Do 5 to 10 repetitions; switch position and repeat; increase until you can do 20.

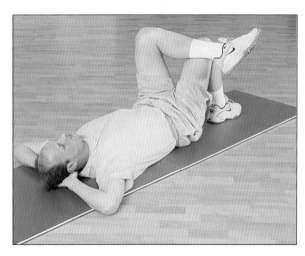 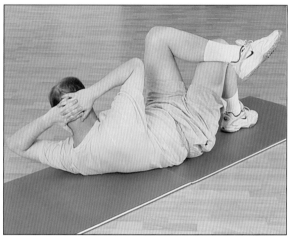

Seated Back Stretch

With your knees bent, bend forward at the waist to bring your head between your knees; pull your abdomen in as you curl forward. Keep your weight back on your hips. Release your abdominal muscles, and reach to stretch your lower back. Come up slowly. Relax; repeat. Move forward to involve and stretch hamstring muscles.

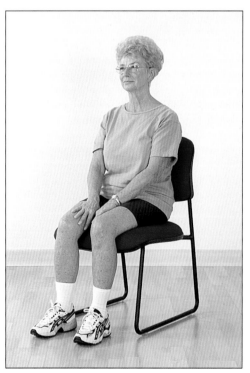 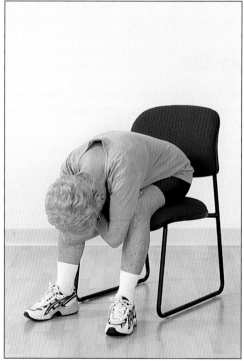

11

Nutrition and Health

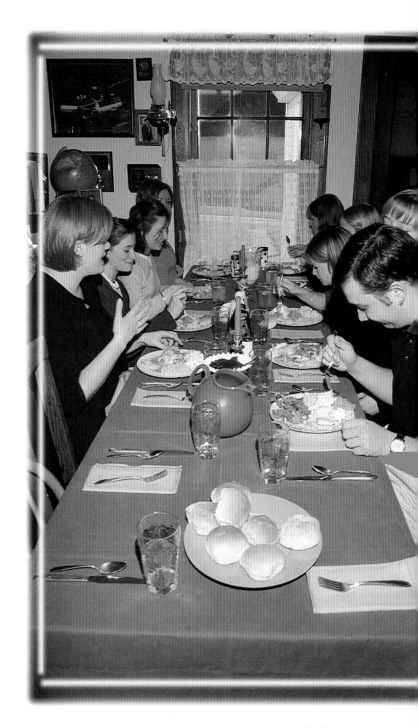

"One must eat to live, and
not live to eat."

Molière

As more people work longer hours, less time is available for the selection and preparation of food, leading to an increasing reliance on prepared food, fast food, ordering in and eating out, and a loss of control over the food we eat. We select the item but have little influence over its preparation. As a consequence, we eat more saturated and hydrogenated fat and more salt, and we run the risk of getting shortchanged in other areas of nutrition.

■ This chapter will help you

- understand the basics of good nutrition,
- identify sources of energy and their contribution to performance and health,
- consider your need for vitamin and mineral supplementation,
- understand the relationship between diet and health, and
- select foods that are good for your health.

Energy

Energy from the sun grows plants that are eaten by animals. Our sources of energy—carbohydrates, fat, and protein—are derived from plant and animal sources. We ingest the food, digest it, and absorb it into the bloodstream for transport to cells. Using enzyme catalysts aligned in metabolic pathways, we convert these energy sources into molecules of ATP (adenosine triphosphate), the high-energy compound responsible for muscular contractions and many other cellular functions. The pathways control the combustion of the fuels that we burn, and we measure energy needs with a unit for measuring heat, the calorie.

The Calorie

A calorie is the amount of heat required to raise one cubic centimeter of water one degree Celsius. The kilocalorie is 1,000 calories, or the heat required to raise one kilogram of water one degree Celsius. Throughout this book, when I talk about calories, I will be referring to the kilocalorie, the standard of measurement in nutrition and exercise.

You always expend some energy, even when you're asleep. If you stay in bed for 24 hours and do nothing at all, you will expend about 1,600 calories (for a 154-pound, or 70-kilogram, body). This energy is used by heart and respiratory muscles, for normal cellular metabolism, and for the maintenance of body temperature. Heavy thinking does little to raise energy needs, but as soon as you begin to move, energy expenditure increases dramatically. Caloric expenditure can go from 1.2 calories per minute at rest to more than 20 calories per minute during vigorous effort. Physical activity has the greatest effect on energy needs. Walking burns about 5 calories per minute, jogging about 10, and running more than 15.

Carbohydrate

Throughout the world carbohydrate provides the major source of energy. It is available in simple and complex forms. Simple sugars such as glucose, fructose, and sucrose (refined sugar composed of molecules of glucose and fructose) contain energy but few nutrients (i.e., vitamins and minerals). Complex carbohy-

On a daily basis:

☐ How many servings of fruits and vegetables do you eat?

☐ How many calories do you consume?

☐ What percentage of your caloric intake comes from fat? From protein? From carbohydrate?

☐ What percentage of each should you get?

☐ What percentage of your fat intake comes from saturated fat?

☐ Do you meet your vitamin and mineral needs?

☐ How many times per week do you eat out, order in, or eat prepared foods?

☐ Do you regularly eat rich sauces, fatty meats, or desserts?

You can evaluate your responses later in this chapter, using information from the section on food choices.

drates found in potatoes, corn, beans, rice, and whole-grained products (bread, pasta) come with important nutrients and fiber. Unfortunately, the average American gets half of his or her dietary carbohydrate from concentrated or refined simple sugars, packed with so-called empty calories (empty because they lack nutrients). Fresh fruits contain simple sugars, but they also provide important nutrients.

Digestion of complex starch molecules begins in the mouth where an enzyme (salivary amalyase) reduces complex carbohydrates to simple sugars. It is temporarily halted in the stomach when the enzyme is inactivated by gastric secretions. In the small intestine, starches are further digested with the help of another enzyme (pancreatic amalyase). Final breakdown to simple sugar form is completed by enzymes secreted by the wall of the intestine. Glucose and other simple sugar molecules are then absorbed into the bloodstream. The absorption is rather complete; most of the sugar you eat gets into the blood, and complex carbohydrates, like potatoes, can enter the blood as quickly as table sugar (Jenkins, Taylor, and Wolever 1982).

The Glycemic Index

Foods that digest rapidly and cause a pronounced rise in blood sugar have a high glycemic index.

The rate of carbohydrate digestion and its effect on the rise of blood glucose is described by the glycemic index. Foods that digest rapidly and cause a pronounced rise in blood sugar have a high glycemic index, whereas those digested and absorbed more slowly, because of fiber or fat, have a low index. As you might expect, foods with a high *glycemic index* include sugar and honey, as well as corn, white bread, refined cereals, and baked potatoes. Moderate–glycemic index foods include pasta, whole-grained breads, rice, oatmeal, bran, and peas; low–glycemic index foods include beans, lentils, and fruits (apples, peaches, grapefruit). High-index foods lead to a rapid rise in blood sugar and a greater rise in insulin, the hormone responsible for lowering blood glucose (Foster-Powell and Miller 1995).

Individuals with insulin resistance, a condition often associated with overweight, hypertension, low HDL-cholesterol, and elevated triglycerides and blood glucose, are wise to select low-index foods. High-index foods prompt an insulin surge from the pancreas, stimulating body cells to store glucose. Over time the cells become less sensitive to insulin, eventually contributing to adult-onset diabetes. Insulin resistance is linked to heart disease, obesity, age, and inactivity. Weight loss and regular moderate activity reduce insulin resistance.

After a meal, absorbed sugars are taken up by the blood, heart, skeletal muscle, and liver, in that order. When blood sugar levels are restored, heart and skeletal muscles accept glucose. The constantly working heart uses it for energy, while the skeletal muscle can store glucose for use when energy is needed. Granules of stored glucose are called muscle glycogen. The liver accepts the simple sugars from the blood and stores them as glycogen. When sufficient glucose has been stored in the liver (about 80 to 100 grams, or 2.8 to 3.5 ounces), the leftover glucose suppresses fat oxidation and is itself used for energy. Thus an excess intake of carbohydrate does not become a supply of "quick energy"; it is oxidized, thereby conserving fat (Swinburn and Ravussin 1993). The glucose stored in the liver is readily available when needed, but muscle glycogen can be used directly only by the muscle in which it is stored. Blood glucose is also used by nerves, muscles, or other tissues in need of energy.

Lactate

Skeletal muscle may convert glucose to lactate, which diffuses from the muscle and travels to the liver for reconversion to glucose, or travels to another muscle for use as a source of energy. In other words, lactate is not just a metabolic by-product, but rather a metabolic intermediate that can shuttle energy from muscle to liver or from muscle to muscle. Oxidative muscle fibers are metabolically suited for lactate oxidation, and endurance training further enhances the fibers' capacity for lactate utilization (Gladden 2000).

Because carbohydrates are important for muscular contractions, and because they are not stored in large quantities, we should consume a sizable percentage of the day's calories from complex carbohydrates and fruit. The performance diet recommended for active people and athletes suggests 55 to 60 percent of the calories from carbohydrates, which is more than the 45 to 50 percent typically consumed (see table 11.1).

As I've noted, carbohydrate is stored in muscles and the liver as granules of glycogen, a compound consisting of many linked molecules of glucose. We use this stored carbohydrate at the start of exercise, and its contribution to energy metabolism increases as exercise intensity increases. During prolonged exercise, when muscle glycogen stores become depleted, we draw on blood glucose that is supplied from the liver stores. When that limited supply runs out, we bonk—a term cyclists coined to describe the utter fatigue, confusion, and lack of coordination that results when blood glucose falls below the level required by the nervous system (see figure 11.1). To avoid bonking, distance athletes consume energy bars

Table 11.1 The Performance Diet

Component	Performance diet (% of total calories)	Typical diet (% of total calories)
Carbohydrate	55-60[a]	45-50
Fat	25-30[b]	35-40
Protein	15	10-15

[a] Increase prior to long distance event (see "Carbohydrate Loading," page 330).
[b] No more than one-third or 33% from saturated or hydrogenated (trans) fats.

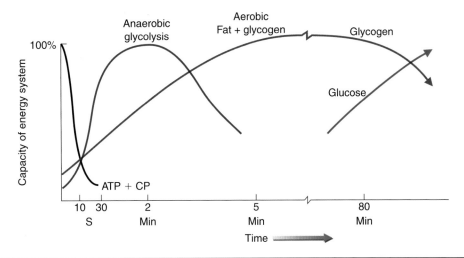

Figure 11.1 Pattern of energy use. We use short-term energy sources (ATP plus CP) at the start of exercise, and then anaerobic or nonoxidative breakdown of glycogen (glycolysis). After several minutes, more efficient aerobic pathways take over, with more carbohydrate use at higher intensities. As muscle glycogen is used up, blood glucose temporarily fills the demand for carbohydrates.

Reprinted from Sharkey 1984.

and drink beverages containing 4 to 10 percent carbohydrate (40 to 100 grams/liter).

Finally, be aware that chronic ingestion of a high-carbohydrate diet—without an active lifestyle—may lead muscle to become insulin insensitive, adipose tissue to convert excess carbohydrate to fat, and the liver to increase production of very low density lipoprotein (VLDL) cholesterol (Graham and Adamo 1999). With regular physical activity, insulin sensitivity is increased, the carbohydrate is burned, and blood lipids are lowered.

Fat

Fat is the most efficient way to store energy, with 9.3 calories per gram versus the 4.1 and 4.3 for carbohydrate and protein, respectively. Dietary fat is broken down and absorbed in the small intestine. It then travels via the lymphatics, a system of tiny vessels and nodes that transport and filter cellular drainage. The fat is eventually dumped into the circulation for transport in clumps (chylomicrons) to cells for energy, or to adipose tissue for storage. However, dietary fat intake isn't

We have many ways to acquire fat but only one good way to remove it: physical activity.

the only way to acquire this source of energy. Excess carbohydrate or protein can be converted to fat and stored in adipose tissue. We have many ways to acquire fat but only one good way to remove it: physical activity.

Fat isn't all bad. It is an essential component of cell walls, vital insulation in the nervous system, a precursor for important compounds such as hormones, and a shock absorber for internal organs. And fat can be a most efficient fuel for sustained physical activity, especially in muscles that have undergone endurance training. Furthermore, fat enhances the taste of food and helps fill us up. So we don't need to eliminate dietary fat, just limit the intake. Excess dietary fat is a major cause of overweight and obesity and a contributor to heart disease, hypertension, diabetes, some cancers, and other ills. And research indicates that a high fat intake is inversely related to physical activity, suggesting a behavioral link between the two (Simoes et al. 1995).

Fat comes in several forms, including triglycerides and cholesterol. Triglyceride fat is composed of three fatty acids and glycerol. The fatty acids can be saturated (with a hydrogen molecule filling each binding site on a carbon molecule) or unsaturated, with one or more double bonds (see figure 11.2).

Monounsaturated fatty acids have one double bond, whereas the polyunsaturated have two or more. The double bonds of unsaturated fatty acids may be more susceptible to oxidation; therefore unsaturated fats are recommended over saturated fats, which facilitate cholesterol synthesis. Saturated fats are found in meat and dairy products. Watch out also for the tropical oils, palm and coconut, which are believed to be more atherogenic (likely to clog arteries), as are some otherwise healthful oils when they are partially hydrogenated (e.g., soybean oil). Hydrogenation eliminates double bonds and creates unhealthy trans fatty acids. Read labels! The performance diet recommends 25 percent of the day's calories from fat, with no more than one-third from saturated (or hydrogenated) fats. This is substantially less than the 35 to 40 percent many people currently consume.

Fat Intake

If you eat 2,000 calories a day and get 25 percent of your calories from fat, you'll get 500 fat calories. Divide 500 by 9.3 calories per gram of fat (500/9.3) and you get 54 grams, the amount of fat you can eat each day (far less than the 86 grams you'd eat if fat constituted 40 percent of your caloric intake). Labels on food packages indicate the grams of fat in each serving.

Cholesterol can be eaten in the diet or synthesized in the liver. Once in the blood it joins with clumps of fat and VLDL. Over a period of two to six hours enzymes remove much of the triglyceride, leaving low-density lipoprotein (LDL) cholesterol, which the liver removes over a period of two to five days. Because of the size of the LDL particle and its high concentration of cholesterol, it finds its way into the walls of coronary arteries and contributes to the development of the atherosclerotic plaque. Thus LDL cholesterol is believed to be a major culprit in the development of coronary artery disease. As LDL levels rise, so does the risk of heart disease (see table 11.2).

High-density lipoprotein (HDL) cholesterol seems to carry cholesterol away from arterial walls to the liver, where it can be removed from the body. This "good" cholesterol has been found to be inversely related to heart disease risk: As

HDL goes up, the risk of coronary artery disease (CAD) goes down! The longitudinal Framingham study of an entire community found HDL to be the single best predictor of heart disease risk. By itself, cholesterol doesn't provide enough information. You need total cholesterol, LDL cholesterol, and HDL cholesterol to assess heart disease risk. And the total cholesterol/HDL ratio may be one of the best ways to assess risk (see table 11.3). I'll say more about the effects of activity and fitness on triglycerides, cholesterol, and heart disease risk in chapter 13.

The fatty acid may be saturated, meaning they have single bonds, such as stearic acid;

Stearic Acid

they may be monounsaturated, meaning they have one double bond, such as oleic acid;

Oleic Acid

or they may be polyunsaturated, meaning they have two or more double bonds, such as linoleic acid.

Linoleic Acid

Figure 11.2 Fatty acids: saturated, monounsaturated, and polyunsaturated.

Table 11.2 Cholesterol Evaluation

	Desirable	Borderline-high	High risk
Cholesterol	<200	200-239	>240 mg/dl*
LDL-C	<130	130-159	>160
HDL-C	>60	59-35	<35

*Milligrams per deciliter (per tenth of a liter); to convert to International System units (millimoles per liter) multiply by 0.0259.

Table 11.3 Total Cholesterol/HDL Ratio

Risk ratio	Male*	Female
0.5	3.43	3.27
1.0	4.97	4.44
2.0	9.55	7.05
3.0	23.4	11.0

*250/50 = 5, an average risk for a male.

Protein

When we ingest animal or plant protein, the large molecules are cleaved into amino acids and absorbed. The amino acids are building blocks used to construct cell walls, muscle tissue, hormones, enzymes, and a variety of other molecules. The blood contains several large proteins: globulin for antibody formation, albumin for buffering and osmosis, fibrinogen for clotting, and hemoglobin for oxygen transport. Training builds proteins; aerobic training builds aerobic enzymes for energy production, and strength training builds contractile proteins (actin and myosin) for strength. So it should be no surprise to learn the importance of protein to the active life.

The performance diet recommends 15 percent of daily caloric intake in the form of protein. Moderately active adults can get by with 10 percent, but we recommend more for those who are very active or training. Fifteen percent of 2,000 calories is 300 calories (300 divided by 4.3 kilocalories per gram equals 70 grams; one gram per kilogram for a person who weighs 70 kilograms, or 154 pounds). More important than quantity, however, is the quality of protein. Quality protein is high in essential amino acids, those that cannot be synthesized in the body. These essential amino acids are macronutrients, major food sources that must be available for optimal function. When essential amino acids are missing, the body is unable to construct proteins that require them. Although animal protein is a better source of essential amino acids (as well as iron and vitamin B12), proper combinations of plant protein can meet nutritional needs. If you are or plan to become a vegetarian, be ready to eat a variety of grains, beans, and leafy vegetables.

> When essential amino acids are missing, the body is unable to construct proteins that require them.

Protein isn't a major source of energy at rest or during exercise—it seldom amounts to more than 5 to 10 percent of energy needs—but when one trains hard while dieting to lose weight, the body senses starvation and begins to use tissue protein for energy. To avoid the loss of muscle tissue and to achieve the benefits of training, ensure adequate protein and energy intake. The best bet is to lose weight slowly or not at all during vigorous training. Even with adequate protein, rapid weight loss while training risks the loss of the muscle and enzyme proteins you are trying so hard to increase.

Protein Needs?

A review of protein needs for athletes concludes that endurance athletes will benefit from dietary intakes of 1.2 to 1.4 grams of protein per kilogram of body weight, and strength athletes need 1.4 to 1.8 grams (Lemon 1995). These values are well above the RDA of 0.8 grams per kilogram but are attainable with the performance diet recommended in this chapter. If you participate in endurance *and* strength training, you'll need at least 1.4 grams per kilogram of body weight. Simply multiply that number times your body weight in kilograms (one kilogram equals 2.2 pounds) to get your daily requirement.

For example, if you weigh 154 pounds, divide 154 by 2.2 to get your weight in kilograms (70). Then multiply 70 times 1.4 grams to get your daily protein needs (in this example, 98 grams). Because each gram of protein yields 4.3 calories, you'll need about 420 (98 grams times 4.3) calories of energy from protein.

Athletes usually raise total caloric intake to meet the increased energy needs of training. If your diet fails to meet the requirements for your type of training, increase your intake of good-quality protein (lean meats, skinned poultry, fish, beans, nuts) (see table 11.4).

Table 11.4 Protein in Common Foods		
Food	**Portion**	**Protein (g)**
Beans	1/2 cup (118 ml)	6-8
Beef	4 ounces (113 g)	20-28
Cheese	1 ounce (28 g)	7
Chicken	3-1/2 ounces (100 g)	24-30
Chili	1 cup (236 ml)	20
Corn	1/2 cup (118 ml)	3
Fish	4 ounces (113 g)	25-30
Hamburger	4 ounces (113 g)	20
Milk	1 cup (236 ml)	9
Peanut butter	1 tablespoon (14 ml)	4
Pizza	1 slice	10

Excess intake of protein, which is often accompanied by fat (e.g., eggs, meat, fish, poultry, dairy products), leads to the storage of energy in the form of fat. Follow the performance diet and you will have all the protein you need, especially since a high carbohydrate intake spares or conserves tissue protein.

Energy Availability

A limited supply of glucose is available in the blood, but it is needed for brain and nerve metabolism, for which it is the sole source of energy. Glucose is stored in the liver (about 80 grams) and muscle (15 grams per kilogram of muscle) as glycogen. If you could use it all for exercise, you would have about 1,200 calories, enough to fuel a 10-mile (16.1-kilometer) run (see table 11.5).

Fat is the most abundant source of energy. Young men average 12.5 percent body fat; young women average 25 percent. If you weigh 121 pounds (55 kilograms) and have 25 percent fat, you'll have about 30 pounds (13.6 kilograms) of fat. Because each pound of fat yields 3,500 calories, 30 pounds of fat provides 105,000 calories of energy. When you consider that you burn about 100 calories per mile (1.6 kilometers) of jogging, you'll realize that you have enough fat energy to fuel 1,000 miles (1,600 kilometers) of running! Most of us have more fat than we need, so you can benefit from teaching the body how to burn fat during exercise. In so doing, you extend your endurance dramatically, eliminate the problem of excess weight, and improve your overall health.

Table 11.5 Available Energy Sources

Source	Supply	Energy (cal)
ATP and CP	Small quantities stored in muscle	5
Carbohydrate		
Muscle glycogen	15 g (per kg of muscle)	1,200
Liver glycogen	80 g	320
Blood glucose	4 g	16
Fat	Adipose tissue	50,000-100,000ª

ªDepends on % body fat and body weight; for example, 15% fat 3 150 lb = 22.5 lb fat; 22.5 lb 3 3,500 cal/lb = 78,750 cal of energy stored as fat.

Adapted from Sharkey 1990.

Nutrients

Sometimes called micronutrients because only small amounts are needed (in contrast to the macronutrients—carbohydrate, fat, and protein), vitamins and minerals play essential roles in metabolism and other important functions.

Vitamins

Why are vitamins, which do not supply energy and are needed only in minute quantities, considered essential for life? In many cases the answer lies in the structure of enzymes that are essential for cellular metabolism. Enzymes are composed of a large protein portion and a coenzyme. The shape of the protein molecule dictates the role of the enzyme, while the coenzyme is the active portion that performs a specific task. For example, vitamin B1 is a coenzyme that removes carbon dioxide in a metabolic pathway. Without the vitamin coenzyme the metabolic pathway grinds to a halt, usually with the toxic buildup of intermediary compounds. Lack of vitamin B1 (thiamine) leads to beriberi, a vitamin deficiency disease characterized by weakness, wasting, nerve damage, and even heart failure. Fortunately, the small amount of vitamins needed are readily available from a variety of foods in a well-balanced diet. Doses far in excess of daily requirements (megadoses) do not improve function or performance, and they may be toxic.

Fortunately, the small amount of vitamins needed are readily available from a variety of foods in a well-balanced diet.

Fat-Soluble Vitamins

Vitamins are classified according to their solubility. The fat-soluble vitamins A, D, E, and K have widely different functions (see table 11.6). These vitamins are ingested with fats in the diet. Amounts in excess of daily needs are stored in body tissue, and megadoses can become toxic (e.g., vitamin A). Because they are stored, deficiencies are less likely, except in very low fat diets.

Water-Soluble Vitamins

B complex vitamins and vitamin C are water-soluble. Excess water-soluble vitamins are flushed away in the urine, making deficiencies more likely. Table 11.6 lists the vitamins along with their recommended daily allowances and good food sources.

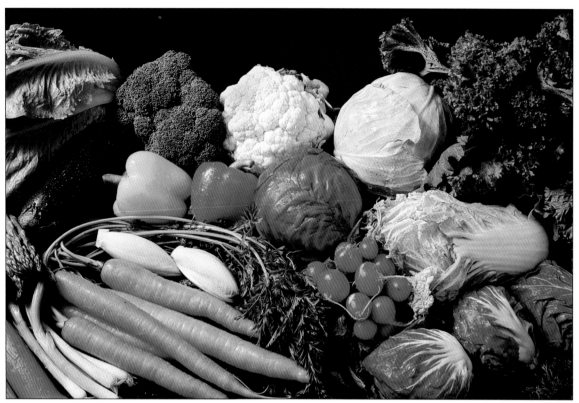

© Kaiser/Photo Network

Vitamins in food have been proven more effective than vitamin supplements.

Vitamins and Health

It is clear that vitamins perform many functions that are essential for life and health. Recent studies indicate that some vitamins are important to the optimal function of the immune system.

To help maintain a healthy immune system, the well-balanced diet should include the following:

- Beta-carotene (carrots, sweet potatoes), which stimulates natural killer cells, immune system cells that fight infections
- Vitamin B6 (potatoes, nuts, spinach), which promotes proliferation of white blood cells
- Folate (peas, salmon, romaine lettuce), which increases white blood cell activity
- Vitamin C (citrus fruits, broccoli, peppers), which enhances the immune response
- Vitamin E (whole grains, wheat germ, vegetable oils), which stimulates the immune response

The minerals selenium and zinc also aid the immune response: Selenium (tuna, eggs, whole grains) promotes action against toxic bacteria, and zinc (eggs, whole grains, oysters) promotes wound healing. Regular moderate physical activity has been found to bolster the immune system, whereas exhaustion and stress impair its function, opening the door to upper respiratory and other infections.

Table 11.6 Vitamins and Minerals: Functions and Sources

Nutrient	Important functions	Sources
Fat-soluble vitamins		
Vit A	Vision, immune function	Milk products
Beta-carotene	Cell growth, antioxidant	Fruits, vegetables
Vit D	Bones, teeth	Sunlight, eggs, fish, milk products
Vit E	Antioxidant	Vegetable oils, nuts, greens
Vit K	Blood clotting	Greens, cereals, fruits, milk products, meats
Water-soluble vitamins		
Vit B_1 (thiamin)	Energy production	Pork, grains, beans
Vit B_2 (riboflavin)	Energy production	Milk, eggs, fish, meat, greens
Niacin	Energy production	Nuts, fish, poultry, grains
Vit B_6 (pyridoxine)	Energy production, protein metabolism	Meats, grains, vegetables, fruits
Folate	Red and white blood cells, RNA, DNA, amino acids	Vegetables, beans, nuts, grains, meat, fruit
Vit B_{12}	Blood cells, RNA, DNA, energy production	Meat, milk products, eggs
Biotin	Fat and amino acid metabolism, glycogen synthesis	Beans, vegetables, meats
Vit C (ascorbic acid)	Wound healing, connective tissue, antioxidant, immune function	Citrus fruits, vegetables
Minerals		
Calcium	Bones, teeth, blood clotting, muscle contraction	Milk products, vegetables, legumes
Chloride	Digestion, extracellular fluids	Salt in food
Chromium	Energy metabolism	Legumes, grains, meats, vegetable oils
Copper	Iron metabolism	Meats, water
Fluorine	Bones, teeth	Water, seafood, tea
Iodine	Thyroid hormone	Fish, milk products, vegetables, salt
Iron	Oxygen transport	Meats, nuts, beans, greens
Magnesium	Protein synthesis	Grains, greens
Phosphorus	Bones, teeth, acid-base balance	Milk products, meats, poultry, fish, grains
Potassium	Nerve transmission, fluid and acid-base balance	Greens, bananas, meats, milk products, potatoes, coffee
Selenium	Antioxidant	Seafood, meats, grain
Sodium	Nerve function, fluid and acid-base balance	Salt
Sulphur	Liver function	Dietary protein
Zinc	Enzyme activity	Meat, poultry, fish, milk products, grains, fruits, vegetables

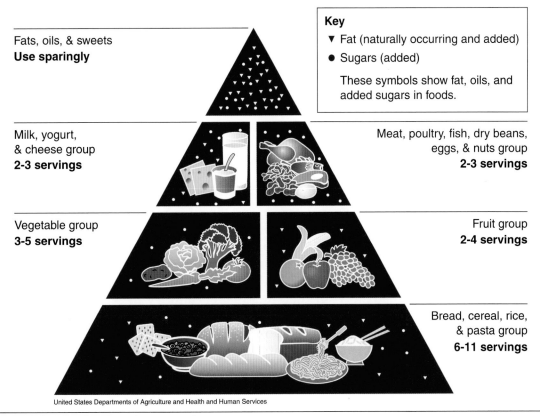

Key

▼ Fat (naturally occurring and added)

● Sugars (added)

These symbols show fat, oils, and added sugars in foods.

Fats, oils, & sweets
Use sparingly

Milk, yogurt,
& cheese group
2-3 servings

Meat, poultry, fish, dry beans,
eggs, & nuts group
2-3 servings

Vegetable group
3-5 servings

Fruit group
2-4 servings

Bread, cereal, rice,
& pasta group
6-11 servings

United States Departments of Agriculture and Health and Human Services

Figure 11.3 The food guide pyramid.

By now it is becoming clear that your diet is an important part of the active life and, along with regular activity, the key to weight control. But is diet related to health for other reasons? Diet has been implicated as a major factor in obesity; heart disease; cancer; diabetes; digestive problems such as diverticulitis, irritable colon, and gallstones; and other problems such as dental carries, hernia, and hemorrhoids. A low-fat diet is prescribed for those at risk for heart disease. But how does diet influence cancer and other problems?

Anticancer Diet

The anticancer diet recently proposed by the National Academy of Sciences endorses the reduction of fat in the diet. The advice includes the following:

Remember, fat is a factor in cancer, heart disease, and diabetes, and exercise is the best way to eliminate excess fat from the body.

- Eat less fat, fatty meats, and dairy products.
- Eat little salt-cured, pickled, or smoked foods.
- Eat more whole-grained products, including fiber-rich foods.
- Eat more fruits and vegetables, including those in the cabbage family and those high in vitamins A and C.
- Drink alcohol in moderation, if at all.
- Keep caloric intake low.

Remember, fat is a factor in cancer, heart disease, and diabetes, and exercise is the best way to eliminate excess fat from the body.

Dietary Fiber

Fiber, roughage, bulk, and bran all refer to the portion of plants that is indigestible. Why consume an indigestible material? In addition to its long-standing reputation for maintaining regularity, fiber has other advantages. Insoluble fiber (wheat bran, beans) holds water, increases bulk, and increases the rate at which stool and cancerous toxins are removed. Soluble fiber, such as oat bran (apples, citrus fruits), forms a gel that slows absorption of carbohydrate and binds cholesterol for removal from the body. It may also produce a chemical that slows the rate of cholesterol production.

Epidemiologic studies show that those on a low-fiber diet have a higher incidence of heart disease, cancer, and the other problems mentioned earlier. The average American consumes about one-third of the 25 to 35 grams (.88 to 1.23 ounces) of fiber recommended by the National Cancer Institute, and the majority regularly ignore fresh fruits and vegetables. If fiber isn't part of your daily regime, begin now to add bran cereals, fruits, vegetables, beans, and whole-grained breads to your diet. Read labels and try to seek a balance between soluble and insoluble fiber. Finally, consider this: When you combine fiber with a low-fat diet and activity, you'll be able to eat freely, with little concern for weight gain (daily activity contributes to regularity and may lower cancer risk by speeding the rate at which stool and toxins pass through the digestive system).

Food, Fitness, and Health

Companies spend millions to convince us that we can achieve fitness and health by eating their products. Though sound nutrition is absolutely essential to health and fitness, nothing you eat will improve your fitness if you are already on an adequate diet. The only way to achieve fitness is via regular exercise; you can't get there just by eating.

Health Foods

Concerns about the quality of our food supply, such as the use of hormones, pesticides, dyes, and other chemicals, has led to wider availability of so-called "health" foods—also known as natural or organic foods—as an alternative source of nutrition. To the extent that these chemicals may be harmful to health, especially over extended periods, natural food sources could be safer. However, the nutritional value of a food or vitamin is not related to the manner of growth. Foods grown with chemical fertilizers are just as nutritious as those grown with organic fertilizers. What matters is the active amount of the essential ingredient, such as a vitamin, and how that contributes to the recommended daily allowance. So purchase more expensive health foods if you are concerned about the effects of chemicals on your health, but don't expect to get super nutrition for the extra expense. Table 11.7 summarizes the recommended dietary allowances (RDA) of proteins, vitamins, and minerals according to age and sex.

Table 11.7 Dietary Reference Intakes and Recommended Dietary Allowances

1997-1998 Dietary Reference Intakes (DRI)

Age (yr)	Recommended Dietary Allowances (RDA)								Adequate Intakes (AI)					
	Thiamin (mg)	Riboflavin (mg)	Niacin (mg NE)	Vitamin B_6 (mg)	Folate (μg DFE)	Vitamin B_{12} (μg)	Phosphorus (mg)	Magnesium (mg)	Vitamin D (μg)	Pantothenic acid (mg)	Biotin (μg)	Choline (mg)	Calcium (mg)	Fluoride (mg)
Infants[a]														
0.0-0.5	0.2	0.3	2[b]	0.1	65	0.4	100	30	5	1.7	5	125	210	0.01
0.5-1.0	0.3	0.4	4	0.3	80	0.5	275	75	5	1.8	6	150	270	0.5
Children														
1-3	0.5	0.5	6	0.6	150	0.9	460	80	5	2.0	8	200	500	0.7
4-8	0.6	0.6	8	0.6	200	1.2	500	130	5	3.0	12	250	800	1.1
Males														
9-13	0.9	0.9	12	1.0	300	1.8	1250	240	5	4.0	20	375	1300	2.0
14-18	1.2	1.3	16	1.3	400	2.4	1250	410	5	5.0	25	550	1300	3.2
19-30	1.2	1.3	16	1.3	400	2.4	700	400	5	5.0	30	550	1000	3.8
31-50	1.2	1.3	16	1.3	400	2.4	700	420	5	5.0	30	550	1000	3.8
51-70	1.2	1.3	16	1.7	400	2.4	700	420	10	5.0	30	550	1200	3.8
>70	1.2	1.3	16	1.7	400	2.4	700	420	15	5.0	30	550	1200	3.8
Females														
9-13	0.9	0.9	12	1.0	300	1.8	1250	240	5	4.0	20	375	1300	2.0
14-18	1.0	1.0	14	1.2	400	2.4	1250	360	5	5.0	25	400	1300	2.9
19-30	1.1	1.1	14	1.3	400	2.4	700	310	5	5.0	30	425	1000	3.1
31-50	1.1	1.1	14	1.3	400	2.4	700	320	5	5.0	30	425	1000	3.1
51-70	1.1	1.1	14	1.5	400	2.4	700	320	10	5.0	30	425	1200	3.1
>70	1.1	1.1	14	1.5	400	2.4	700	320	15	5.0	30	425	1200	3.1
Pregnancy	1.4	1.4	18	1.9	600	2.6	*	+40	*	6.0	30	450	*	*
Lactation	1.5	1.6	17	2.0	500	2.8	*	*	*	7.0	35	550	*	*

(continued)

Table 11.7 (continued)

1989 Recommended Dietary Allowances (RDA)

Age (yr)	Energy (kcal)	Protein (g)	Vitamin A (μg RE)	Vitamin E (mg α-TE)	Vitamin K (μg)	Vitamin C (mg)	Iron (mg)	Zinc (mg)	Iodine (μg)	Selenium (μg)
Infants										
0.0-0.5	650	13	375	3	5	30	6	5	40	10
0.5-1.0	850	14	375	4	10	35	10	5	50	15
Children										
1-3	1300	16	400	6	15	40	10	10	70	20
4-6	1800	24	500	7	20	45	10	10	90	20
7-10	2000	28	700	7	30	45	10	10	120	30
Males										
11-14	2500	45	1000	10	45	50	12	15	150	40
15-18	3000	59	1000	10	65	60	12	15	150	50
19-24	2900	58	1000	10	70	60	10	15	150	70
25-50	2900	63	1000	10	80	60	10	15	150	70
51+	2300	63	1000	10	80	60	10	15	150	70
Females										
11-14	2200	46	800	8	45	50	15	12	150	45
15-18	2200	44	800	8	55	60	15	12	150	50
19-24	2200	46	800	8	60	60	15	12	150	55
25-50	2200	50	800	8	65	60	15	12	150	55
51+	1900	50	800	8	65	60	10	12	150	55
Pregnancy	+300	60	800	10	65	70	30	15	175	65
Lactation										
1st 6 mo.	+500	65	1300	12	65	95	15	19	200	75
2nd 6 mo.	+500	62	1200	11	65	90	15	16	200	75

*Values for these nutrients do not change with pregnancy or lactation. Use the value listed for women of comparable age.

aFor all nutrients, an AI was established instead of an RDA as the goal for infants; for the B vitamins and choline, the age groupings are 0 through 5 months and 6 through 11 months.

bThe AI for niacin for this age group only is stated as milligrams of preformed niacin instead of niacin equivalents.

Reprinted from National Academy of Sciences 1999.

Energy in Foods

How is the energy or caloric value of food determined? Nutrition researchers use a calorimeter to measure the energy content of foods. A small amount of food is placed in a chamber and burned in the presence of oxygen. The heat liberated in the process indicates the energy content of the food (one kilocalorie is the heat required to raise one kilogram of water one degree Celsius). When a gram of carbohydrate is ignited, the energy yield is 4.1 kilocalories. When fat is tested, more than twice as much energy is released (see table 12.1).

Table 12.1 Caloric Equivalents of Foods

Food	Energy (cal/g)[a]	Oxygen (L/g)	Caloric equivalent (cal/L)
Fat	9.3	1.98	4.696
Carbohydrate	4.1	0.81	5.061
Protein	4.3	0.97	4.432

The alcohol in alcoholic beverages has a high caloric value, 7.1 cal/g. The calories are "empty" and provide no nutritional value. Moreover, because alcohol diminishes appetite and interferes with digestion by inflammation of the stomach, pancreas, and intestine, alcohol often leads to malnutrition. Alcohol also interferes with vitamin activation by the liver and causes liver damage (Lieber 1976).

[a]Cal (kilocalories) refers to the amount of heat energy required to raise the temperature of 1 kg of water 1°C.

Reprinted from Sharkey 1974.

Energy Expenditure

You always expend some energy, even when you are asleep. But when you begin to move, energy needs increase dramatically. Energy expenditure can go from 1.2 calories per minute during rest to more than 20 calories per minute during vigorous activity. Energy is also needed when you eat to power the processes of digestion and absorption. But it is physical activity that has the greatest effect on energy expenditure. Walking involves an expenditure of about 5 calories per minute, jogging burns 10 or more, and running can expend 15 to 20 calories per minute (see figure 12.1).

In the fasted state (12 hours after last meal), fat, including plasma free fatty acids (plasma FFA) and muscle triglyceride, is the predominate source of energy at light and moderate levels of exercise intensity. At higher levels, carbohydrate, in the form of muscle glycogen and blood glucose, becomes the major fuel. The contribution of carbohydrate would be somewhat higher during moderate exercise following a high-carbohydrate meal. The relative contribution of each fuel changes throughout several hours of continuous exercise. For example, at 75 percent of $\dot{V}O_2$max, the contribution of muscle glycogen drops from 45 percent to near zero upon depletion of the supply, while energy derived from muscle triglyceride declines from 25 to 10 percent. The role of blood glucose increases from 5 to 40 percent as muscle glycogen is depleted. But when the liver glycogen

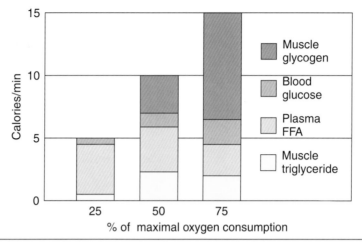

Figure 12.1 Sources of energy. Approximate contribution of energy sources at three levels of exercise. Plasma free fatty acids (FFA) are transported via the blood to the muscles.

percent of $\dot{V}O_2$max, the contribution of muscle glycogen drops from 45 percent to near zero upon depletion of the supply, while energy derived from muscle triglyceride declines from 25 to 10 percent. The role of blood glucose increases from 5 to 40 percent as muscle glycogen is depleted. But when the liver glycogen supply declines, the blood glucose falls precipitiously. The contribution of fat from adipose tissue (plasma FFA) increases throughout prolonged exercise, rising from 25 to 50 percent after several hours (Coyle 1995).

Your energy expenditure depends on the size of your body.

Your energy expenditure depends on the size of your body. The greater the body weight, the higher the caloric expenditure. The caloric expenditure tables in this book are based on a body weight of about 70 kilograms (154 pounds). If you weigh 7 kilograms (about 15 pounds) more, add 10 percent; if you weigh 7 kilograms less, subtract 10 percent; and so forth. For example, if you weigh 124 pounds (56.2 kilograms) and the caloric cost of slow jogging is listed at 10 calories per minute, subtract 20 percent, or 2 calories, to find the calories burned when you jog (8 calories per minute).

Exercise and Weight Control

Some types of exercise are better than others for weight control. As you know, we shift from fat to carbohydrate metabolism as exercise becomes more vigorous. If

Table 12.2 Physical Activity and Caloric Expenditure

Work intensity	Pulse rate	Expenditure (cal/min)	Examples
Light	Below 120	Under 5	Golf, bowling, walking, volleyball, most work
Moderate[a]	120-150	5 to 10	Jogging, tennis, bike riding, aerobic dance, basketball, hiking, racquetball, strenuous work
Heavy	Above 150	Above 10	Running; fast swimming; other brief, intense efforts

[a]Preferred for weight-control benefits
Reprinted from Sharkey 1974.

desire to burn excess fat, consider moderate exercise (see table 12.2). Because extremely vigorous activity cannot be sustained for very long, the total caloric expenditure may not be great. Also, fat utilization increases over time, with more fat being burned after 30 minutes of exercise. Moderate activity can be continued for hours without undue fatigue, thereby allowing a significant fat metabolism and caloric expenditure.

Incidentally, while we are on the subject of fat metabolism, the best time to exercise for weight control may be in the morning, before breakfast, when you are more likely to burn fat after an overnight fast. So if you are interested in fat metabolism and weight control, try morning exercise. However, if it doesn't suit your biological clock, don't despair. Exercise always burns calories, so it always contributes to weight control.

Measuring Energy Expenditure

In the early part of this century, scientists found a way to measure human energy expenditure. Subjects were placed in a double-walled chamber very much like a calorimeter. Heat generated in physical activity eventually increased the temperature of the water layer surrounding the chamber, indicating the caloric (heat) expenditure. However, this method was far too expensive, time-consuming, and cumbersome for the measurement of vigorous activity. Drawing on their knowledge concerning the oxygen requirements of metabolism, researchers developed indirect methods of calorimetry. Because each liter of oxygen consumed is equivalent to about five calories, why not just measure the oxygen used during exercise? The closed-circuit method of indirect calorimetry still is used in hospitals, usually for resting or basal metabolic studies. The amount of oxygen taken from a large tank is measured directly.

The open-circuit method is best suited for vigorous exercise. The subject breathes readily available atmospheric air, and the exhaled air is collected for analysis. The oxygen consumed and carbon dioxide produced during the activity are analyzed, along with the total volume of exhaled air. Oxygen consumption per minute is simply:

(Atmospheric oxygen – Exhaled oxygen) × Volume exhaled air

(20.93% – 17.93%) × 33.3 liters = 1.0 liter oxygen per minute

One liter of oxygen equals about 5 calories per minute, the energy cost of a brisk walk. Jogging requires two liters per minute, or about 10 calories.

It is easy to do metabolic conversions, or convert from total calories to calories per minute (cal/min) to oxygen equivalents in liters (L/min) or milliliters (ml/kg · min) to metabolic equivalents (METs) (see figure 12.2).

Figure 12.2 To convert from one unit to another, simply carry out the calculation in the direction indicated by the arrow. For example, if you use one liter of oxygen per minute (1 L/min) in a brisk walk, you'll burn five calories per minute (1 L times 5 equals 5 calories per minute) and 300 calories per hour (5 times 60).

Energy Balance

Energy balance refers to a comparison between energy intake, the calories consumed in the diet, and energy expenditure, the calories burned in the course of all daily activities (see figure 12.3). If intake exceeds expenditure, the excess will be stored as fat. Since the 1960s Americans have reduced total dietary fat intake from 40 percent to about 35 percent of daily calories. Unfortunately, we've

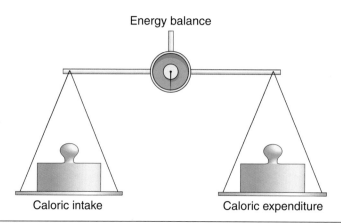

Figure 12.3 Energy balance.

One pound (.45 kilogram) of body fat has the energy equivalent of 3,500 calories. Therefore, about 3,500 calories must be expended (oxidized or burned) to remove one pound of stored fat. Conversely, 3,500 calories of excess dietary intake will lead to an additional pound of body weight. For example, the daily activity of a young man whose body weight is around 70 kilograms (154 pounds) consists of light office work. He does not engage in any physical activity, so his daily caloric needs approximate 2,400 calories. If he eats a sweet roll for an additional 250 calories on a daily basis, what will happen to him over the course of one year?

250 calories × 30 days per month = 7,500 calories × 12 = 90,000 calories per year

That 90,000 calories he has gained divided by 3,500 calories per pound equates to 25.7 pounds (11.7 kilograms) of added weight. No wonder 33 percent of the population is overweight. Our friend has upset his energy balance to the tune of more than 2 pounds (.9 kilogram) per month, or 25.7 pounds per year. If he does nothing about his diet or exercise, he could gain 257 pounds (116.5 kilograms) in 10 years! Of course, the reverse is also true. If he gives up (or burns) 250 calories each day, he could lose more than 25 pounds a year. One purpose of this book is to teach you how to have your cake and eat it too, how to use diet and exercise to achieve control of your weight.

Caloric Intake

Determining your caloric intake is the first step in calculating your energy balance. Table 12.3 includes comprehensive calorie charts organized according to general categories (e.g., vegetables, meat). Calories contained in each portion are given. Remember these conversions (English-to-metric conversions are listed below the English conversions):

- 3 teaspoons = 1 tablespoon
- 2 tablespoons = 1 fluid ounce
- 16 tablespoons = 1 cup
- 1 cup = 8 fluid ounces, or one-half pint
- 4 cups = 1 quart
- 1 pound = 16 ounces

- 1 tablespoon = 14.8 milliliters
- 1 fluid ounce = 29.6 milliliters
- 1 cup = 237 milliliters, or .24 liter
- 1 quart = .95 liter
- 1 pound = 453.6 grams, or .45 kilogram

Determine your daily caloric intake by keeping an accurate account of everything you eat and drink. The most accurate picture comes when you keep records for several days. Record the food or drink and the amount actually consumed. Then use table 12.3 to determine your caloric intake. For example, breakfast consists of one cup of corn flakes (100 calories) with one-half cup skim milk (40), sugar (25), and a sliced banana (94), plus two pieces of toast (110) with butter (20) and jelly (50), and black coffee (1). Total caloric intake is 440 calories. Do the same for all meals, snacks, beverages . . . everything. Add up the day's total, and that is your caloric intake. If it regularly exceeds your daily caloric expenditure, you will gain weight. See figure 12.4 on page 250 for a sample worksheet.

Carry a small notepad with you so that you can jot down any food, drink, or snack consumed. At the end of the day sit down with the calorie charts and figure your daily intake. Computer programs are available to simplify the calculations and provide information on the nutritional value of your diet. You should attempt to assess your caloric intake for several typical days; it is a most educational experience.

Table 12.3 also includes the grams of fat contained in each portion of food or beverage. This should help you avoid high-fat foods if you decide to pursue a low-fat diet, which helps to reduce body weight and blood lipids. Each gram of fat contains 9.3 calories. If your goal is to reduce fat intake from the typical 40 percent of calories, try to stay within the following targets:

For a daily caloric intake of 2,000 calories:

40% fat = 86 grams of fat

(40% × 2,000 calories = 800 calories / 9.3 cal / gm = 86 grams of fat)

30% fat = 65 grams

20% fat = 43 grams

10% fat = 22 grams

Caloric Expenditure

For the next few days, keep an inventory of your activity. Simply list your activity (exercise, work, household chores) and the time spent for each (see figure 12.5 on page 251). Don't omit anything, even sleeping. This inventory exercise is very educational; it shows you when calories are burned and provides insight about how you can increase caloric expenditures in your normal routine.

Then estimate the caloric expenditure by referring to the caloric expenditure tables (tables 12.4 and 12.5 on page 252) and to figure 12.6 on page 253. I've provided two ways to estimate your caloric expenditure, one short and one long. The long method requires that you keep records of your daily activities: sleep, dressing, cooking, work, and all physical activity, including walking, stair climbing, fitness, and recreation.

Table 12.3 Caloric Content of Foods

Food	Portion	Fat[a] (grams)	Calories
Beverages, alcoholic			
Beer	12 ounces (355 ml)	0	150
Beer, light	12 ounces (355 ml)	0	100
Brandy	1 ounce (30 ml)	0	70
Eggnog	8 ounces (240 ml)	19	335
Highball	8 ounces (240 ml)	0	165
Port, vermouth, muscatel	4 ounces (120 ml)	0	155
Rum	1 jigger (1-1/2 ounces) (44 ml)	0	140
Whiskey	1 jigger (1-1/2 ounces) (44 ml)	0	130
Wine, white, rosé	4 ounces (120 ml)	0	85-105
Beverages, nonalcoholic			
Carbonated soft drinks	8 ounces (240 ml)	0	80
Chocolate milk	8 ounces (240 ml)	10.5	200
Cocoa	8 ounces (240 ml)	11	75
Coffee, black	8 ounces (240 ml)	0	1
with cream and sugar (1 teaspoon each)	8 ounces (240 ml)	3	45
Tea	8 ounces (240 ml)	0	1
Cereals, cereal products			
Bread			
Boston, enriched, brown	2 large slices	1.2	200
corn or muffins, enriched	2	6	220
raisin, enriched	2 slices	1.5	130
rye, American	2 slices	0.6	110
white, enriched	2 slices	1.5	120
whole wheat	2 slices	1.5	110
Bread, rolls, sweet, unenriched	1	3	320
Cornflakes	1 cup (240 ml)	0.1	100
Crackers, graham	2	1.0	60
saltines	2	1.5	50
soda	10 oyster	1.3	40
Macaroni, cooked	1/2 cup (120 ml)	0.3	70
Noodles, cooked	1 cup (240 ml)	2.0	150
Oatflakes, cooked	1 cup (240 ml)	1.0	75
Pancakes, wheat	2 cakes	6.0	150

Food	Portion	Fat[a] (grams)	Calories
Cabbage, fresh	wedge	0.2	25
Carrots, canned	1/2 cup (120 ml)	0.2	30
fresh	1 carrot (6 in.)	0.1	20
Cauliflower, fresh	1 cup (240 ml)	0.2	25
Celery	2 stalks	0.1	17
Corn, fresh, with butter	1 ear	2.0	90
canned	1/2 cup (120 ml)	0.6	70
Cucumbers	1 (7-1/2 in.)	0.2	20
Eggplant, fresh	1/2 cup (120 ml)	0.2	25
Kale, fresh	1/2 cup (120 ml)	0.4	20
Lentils	1/2 cup (120 ml)	—	110
Lettuce, headed, fresh	1/4 head	0.1	15
Mushrooms	1/2 cup (120 ml)	0.1	10
Onions	1 (2-1.2 in.)	0.1	40
Peas, green, fresh	1/2 cup (120 ml)	0.2	55
canned	1/2 cup (120 ml)	0.4	70
Peppers, green, fresh	1 large	0.1	24
Potatoes, raw	1 medium	0.2	90
French fried	20 pieces	12	220
Radishes, fresh	4 small	—	10
Rhubarb, fresh	1/2 cup (120 ml)	—	10
Spinach, canned	1/2 cup (120 ml)	0.2	25
Sweet potatoes, fresh	1 small	0.6	150
candied	1 medium	3.5	180
Tomatoes, fresh	1 medium	0.2	25
canned	1/2 cup (120 ml)	0.2	25
Tomato juice, canned	4 ounces (114 g)	0.2	35
Miscellaneous			
Gelatin dessert	4 ounces (114 g)	0	60
Pie	1 slice	16-18	300-400
Pecan pie	1 slice	31.5	580
Potato chips	7-10	8.0	110
Salad dressing (French, Thousand Island)	1 tablespoon (15 ml)	6-8	60-100
Tomato catsup	2 tablespoons (30 ml)	0.1	40
Yeast, compressed, baker's	1 cake	0.1	20

[a]1 g of fat contains 9.3 calories

Caloric Intake Record

(Use calorie charts in table 12.3.)

Date _____   Weight _____

	Food	Portion	Intake (cal)
Breakfast			
Lunch			
Dinner			
Desserts			
Snacks			
Drinks			
Other			
Total caloric intake			_____
Total caloric expenditure (figure 12.5)			_____

Energy balance (+ or -) _____

Cal/day

Figure 12.4   Caloric intake record.

When intake and expenditure have been determined, you will be able to assess your energy balance, and you'll have a clear idea of what you can do to reduce caloric intake and increase caloric expenditure.

Short Method

Follow steps 1 through 4:

1. Calculate basal energy expenditure using table 12.4.

2. Add increases in caloric expenditure using table 12.5.

3. Adjust total for age: subtract 4 percent of caloric expenditure for each decade (10 years) over 25 years of age.

4. Add calories expended in nonwork (recreational) activities.

Use the caloric expenditure charts in figure 12.6 to calculate minutes of activity and cost in calories per minute.

Example: A 45-year-old construction worker, 5 feet 10 inches tall, weighing 200 pounds (91 kilograms)

Basal = 1,815 calories + 100%

= 3,630 calories – 8% (age)

= 3,340 calories + 30 minutes of table tennis with his son (30 minutes × 5 calories per minute)

= 150 calories

Total = 3,490 calories per day

Caloric Expenditure Log

(Use energy expenditure tables in this chapter.)

Activity	Time (min)	Expenditure rate (cal/min)	Total expenditure (cal)
Sleep	_____	_____	_____
Nonwork and household			
_____	_____	_____	_____
_____	_____	_____	_____
_____	_____	_____	_____
Work			
_____	_____	_____	_____
_____	_____	_____	_____
_____	_____	_____	_____
Recreation and sport			
_____	_____	_____	_____
_____	_____	_____	_____
_____	_____	_____	_____
	24 hr	Day's total =	_____

Examples	Time (min)	Expenditure rate (cal/min)	Total expenditure (cal)
Sleep	480	1.2	576
Nonwork			
Personal toilet	10	2.0	20
Cook breakfast	10	1.5	15
Cook dinner	60	1.5	90
TV/read	210	1.5	315
Visit	60	2.0	120
Shop	50	3.0	150
Work			
Walk to work and return	20	5.0	100
Work (standard activity)	400	2.6	1,040
Rest breaks	80	1.5	120
Lunch	30	1.5	45
Jogging	30	10.0	300
			Total 2,891

Figure 12.5 Caloric expenditure log.

Table 12.4 Basal Energy Expenditure for Men and Women

Men		Women	
Weight	Energy expenditure[a] (cal)	Weight	Energy expenditure[b] (cal)
140 (64 kg)	1,550	100 (45 kg)	1,225
160 (73 kg)	1,640	120 (54 kg)	1,320
180 (82 kg)	1,730	140 (64 kg)	1,400
200 (91 kg)	1,815	160 (73 kg)	1,485
220 (100 kg)	1,900	180 (82 kg)	1,575

[a]5 ft 10 in. (1.8 m) tall (add 20 cal for each inch taller; if shorter subtract 20 cal for each inch).

[b]5 ft 6 in. (1.7 m) tall (add 20 cal for each inch taller; if shorter subtract 20 cal for each inch).

Basal energy = calories expended in 24 hr of complete bed rest.

Table 12.5 Approximate Increases in Caloric Expenditure for Selected Activities

Activity	Percent above basal
Bed rest (eating and reading)	10
Quiet sitting (reading, knitting)	30
Light activity (office work)	40-60
Moderate activity (housekeeping)	60-80
Heavy occupational activity (construction)	100

Long Method

You calculated your daily caloric expenditure using the short method. This section provides the information for a minute-by-minute estimation of caloric expenditure that allows the computation of a 24-hour total. You may be interested in comparing the two methods to see if they agree. If so, begin by making a list of your daily activities. Then proceed to determine the cost of each activity in calories per minute. Finally, get the total for each activity and the total for the day. Figure 12.6 shows how this can be done.

Table 12.6, which shows caloric expenditure, also serves as a useful guide to exercise intensity because intensity is directly related to calories expended per minute. The caloric expenditure charts can guide you to appropriate weight-control activities. You can readily see that walking burns more calories than recreational volleyball, running more calories than calisthenics. And the charts will tell you how long you should exercise to burn a specific number of calories (e.g., 10 calories per minute for 10 minutes will burn 100 calories).

Be sure to adjust the totals for your body weight: Add 10 percent for each 15 pounds (6.8 kilograms) above 150 pounds (68 kilograms), and subtract 10 percent for each 15 pounds below 150 pounds.

Your energy balance can now be calculated as follows:

Caloric intake = ___ calories — Caloric expenditure = ___ calories

Table 12.8 Minimum Thickness of Triceps Indicating Obesity

Age	Male (mm)	Female (mm)
5	12	14
10	16	20
15	16	24
20	16	28
25	20	29
30-50	23	30

Obesity is defined as more than 20% fat for men; more than 30% fat for women.

Adapted from Seltzer and Mayer 1965.

You should strive to remain at or near the desirable category; heavier men and women in all age groups have an increased risk of death from all causes.

sure fat. New methods of estimating fat are often compared with underwater weighing to see if they are accurate. However, recent studies indicate that underwater weighing itself is subject to errors, especially with younger and older subjects and those at the extremes of leanness and fatness (Going 1996). Age-related differences in body water and bone density can throw off this method, as can dehydration. Therefore, studies are under way to improve the equations used to calculate body fat from underwater weighing. Until then, skinfolds, girth measurements (figure 12.9), or the body mass index (figure 12.10) can guide your weight-control efforts.

The body mass index (BMI), defined as weight in kilograms divided by height in meters squared, provides a simple way for you to assess body composition. Look at figure 12.10 to assess your BMI. All you need is your body weight in pounds and your height in inches. Then use figure 12.10 to get your score. You should strive to remain at or near the desirable category; heavier men and women in all age groups have an increased risk of death from all causes (Calle et al. 1999). However, it is also true that low fitness is an independent predictor of mortality in all body mass index groups, and the risks of being overweight are much lower in those who maintain a higher level of aerobic fitness (Wei et al. 1999).

Getting Fat

Excess caloric intake starts the process. Fat intake poses more of a problem, though, because it has 9.3 calories per gram, whereas carbohydrate and protein have 4.1 and 4.3 calories per gram, respectively. Moreover, fat is similar to the composition of our adipose tissue and easier to store. Obese people eat more fat and engage in less physical activity (Rising et al. 1994), thereby contributing to the problem. Some researchers believe fat cells may continue to increase in size and number in severely obese individuals with increasing food intake, creating an even greater urge to eat. Rising obesity increases levels of the enzyme lipoprotein lipase (LPL), which helps fat cells take on more fat. Excess fat seems to inhibit the action of insulin, the hormone that helps glucose get into cells, leading to feelings of weakness and hunger that cause one to eat more. And the cycle continues.

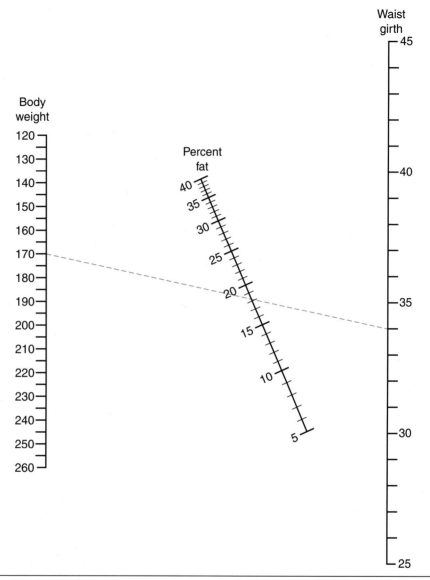

Figure 12.9 Girth measurements. Various body dimensions have been used to predict lean body weight and percent fat. For men only, the girth at the waist seems to be a good predictor of body fat. For this method simply measure the girth of the waist at the level of the navel, then use a straight edge and go from waist girth to body weight to estimate percent fat. For other tape measure methods to estimate body fat consult McArdle, Katch, and Katch (1994).

Reprinted from Sharkey 1990.

Causes of Overweight and Obesity

Why are 80 million Americans overweight to the point of obesity? Is it merely because their caloric intake exceeds expenditure? To a large extent, the answer is yes! Although Americans have lowered the proportion of fat in their diet, they have simultaneously increased carbohydrate and caloric intake and decreased their level of physical activity. However, scientists continue to study other possible contributions to the epidemic of obesity.

food intake, but the appetite doesn't keep pace with energy output. Regular activity seems to help the appestat adjust caloric intake to energy needs. The appestat is rather imprecise at a low level of energy expenditure, but for regularly active individuals, appetite control is much more related to energy needs (Mayer and Bullen 1974). And at the high end of the activity scale, where endurance athletes and workers burn 4,000 to 6,000 calories daily in running, cycling, swimming, or work, the appetite usually underestimates energy needs (Ruby, Schoeller, and Sharkey 2001).

Psychological factors such as the smell, sight, or taste of food can evoke the desire to eat. Habit and emotional factors also condition eating behavior. We eat to celebrate, to prolong feelings of excitement. Appetite is a complex phenomenon, subject to many influences, reflecting more than the need for nourishment. The appestat frequently overestimates energy needs. Weight control becomes possible when you realize that your eyes are bigger than your stomach and your potential for energy intake is greater than your regular energy expenditure.

Premeal or Postmeal Exercise

Years ago, when the American diet was first implicated as a culprit in the heart disease epidemic, researchers roamed the world studying the relationship between diet and the incidence of heart disease. They found that diet alone did not account for the presence or absence of the problem; other factors such as a lack of tension and stress or physical activity confounded the relationship. Several researchers have focused on the effect of pre- or postmeal exercise on postprandial lipemia, the presence of fat in the blood after a meal. Studies conducted at the University of Florida have shown that exercise before or after a meal is effective in reducing the magnitude and duration of postprandial lipemia (Zauner, Burt, and Mapes 1968). Mild exercise proved to be as effective as strenuous effort in this regard.

Activity Versus Caloric Restriction

Recent research indicates that the effect of exercise on postprandial lipid lipemia is greater than and different from the effect attributable to a comparable caloric deficit. A 90-minute walk reduced postprandial lipemia 20 percent below control levels, whereas caloric restriction reduced it only 7 percent (Gill and Hardman 2000).

Lipemia has long been associated with atherosclerosis, reduced myocardial blood flow, and accelerated blood clotting. Thus anything that reduces the level of fat in the blood seems prudent and advisable. Vigorous premeal exercise may inhibit the appetite and increase the metabolism of fat, even fat ingested after the exercise. The metabolic rate remains somewhat elevated after exercise, and the ingested fat is used quickly to restore energy burned during exercise. Mild postmeal effort such as a walk after dinner also serves to reduce lipemia. Both pre- and postmeal exercise increase caloric expenditure and fat metabolism, lead to improved fitness, and contribute to health and weight control.

And, while we're on the subject of meals and blood lipids, you should know that the number of meals you eat has an influence on blood fat levels. Spread the same number of calories over more meals (three to six), and cholesterol levels will be lower. Presumably we are able to handle fat better in smaller doses. Conversely, if you avoid meals in an effort to lose weight, your metabolic rate will decline and your cholesterol level will climb. And your temporary weight loss may be followed by a rapid gain.

Fitness and Fat

The effects of activity on weight control and energy balance are well established. When the exercise is systematic and progressive, it leads to an improvement in aerobic fitness. This section deals with the extra benefits associated with improved fitness, benefits that provide dramatic evidence of the role fitness plays in health and the prevention of heart disease. These benefits include the following:

- Increased caloric expenditure
- Increased fat mobilization
- Increased fat utilization
- Reduced blood lipids
- Increased lean tissue (muscle)

Caloric Expenditure

Unfit individuals tire quickly during exercise and are limited in their ability to expend calories. As fitness improves, caloric expenditure increases with increases in the intensity, duration, and frequency of exercise and because of the inevitable participation in more vigorous activities. The fit individual does more with less fatigue. Thus increased fitness undoubtedly contributes to energy expenditure and weight control.

We studied the effects of training on individuals' perception of effort and fatigue (Docktor and Sharkey 1971). As fitness improved, more work could be performed at the same heart rate and level of perceived exertion. Work levels once perceived as difficult became less so, and once-fatiguing exertion could be managed with ease. After training, a given task could be accomplished with a lower heart rate as well as a lower level of perceived exertion. Thus the subjects were able to burn more energy without experiencing a greater sense of fatigue.

Further proof of the value of fitness to caloric expenditure is found in the relationship of caloric expenditure to heart rate. Caloric expenditure is related directly to the heart rate, but the relationship is also influenced by level of fitness. For people in low fitness categories, a high heart rate does not indicate an extremely high caloric expenditure (see figure 13.1). For those in high fitness categories, the same heart rate (HR) indicates a much higher energy expenditure:

140 HR for the very poor fitness level = 6 to 7 calories per minute expended

140 HR for the very good fitness level = 12 calories per minute expended

You can use figure 13.1 to estimate your caloric expenditure in any activity. After several minutes of participation, stop and immediately take your pulse at wrist or throat (use gentle contact) for 15 seconds. Multiply by four to get your rate per minute. Then use the line corresponding to your fitness level to estimate your caloric expenditure per minute. Also notice how caloric expenditure will improve (at the same heart rate) as your fitness improves. This should convince you that fitness provides extra benefits to those who persevere.

group, while total cholesterol was only "modestly" reduced. However, when the lipoprotein pattern was analyzed, the joggers exhibited a significantly lower level of dangerous LDL and an elevated level of high-density lipoprotein (HDL). These findings were significant, because there is a direct relationship between LDL and heart disease and an inverse relationship between HDL and heart disease (as HDL goes up, the incidence of heart disease goes down). HDL seems to carry cholesterol away from the tissues for removal by the liver. Dr. Wood noted that the lipoprotein pattern of the active men could be mistaken for that of the typical young woman, who has the lowest risk of heart disease in the adult population.

When researchers studied the effects of seven weeks of training on the serum lipids and lipoproteins in 13 young medical students, triglycerides were reduced (from 110 to 80 milligrams) (Lopez et al. 1974). Furthermore, they found a marked reduction of beta lipoprotein cholesterol (cholesterol in LDL and VLDL), a concomitant increase in alpha lipoprotein cholesterol (HDL), and no changes in body weight to confuse the results. Studies in our lab (Sharkey et al. 1980) agree with those reported by Dr. Wood and many others. They clearly indicate how training helps shift cholesterol from the dangerous LDL to the favorable HDL, why total cholesterol fails to indicate all the effects of exercise, and how activity and fitness help reduce the risk of coronary artery disease.

How's that for an extra benefit of fitness? Not only does fitness allow increased caloric expenditure and enhanced fat mobilization and utilization, but it also allows you to have a direct effect on the blood lipids and reduce your risk of heart disease. In my view, this may be the most important benefit of exercise and fitness. If all this doesn't convince you to become active and improve your aerobic fitness . . . I'll just have to keep trying.

One final word to keep your interest. There is a growing belief among researchers in this area that it may be possible to lower serum cholesterol levels enough to actually reverse the process of atherosclerosis, to remove fatty buildup from the lining of the coronary arteries. If it proves to be true that diet and exercise, perhaps with the help of drug therapy, can accomplish this reversal, it will be possible to cure, not just treat, many cases of the nation's number-one killer.

Lean Tissue

Finally, let me remind you that muscle is the furnace that burns fat. Whereas dieting leads to a loss of muscle, a lower metabolic rate, and a reduced ability to exercise and burn fat, fitness training has the capacity to maintain or increase muscle mass and burn more calories and more fat. Aerobic training such as running leads to a small increase in lean body weight. Training with more resistance, such as in cycling, can cause more noticeable changes in muscle. And, of course, muscular fitness (resistance) training leads to impressive changes in muscle mass. Fortunately, muscle lost in dieting can be rapidly reclaimed with activity and training.

Whereas aerobic exercise doesn't have a great effect on the resting metabolic rate, resistance training has been shown to increase strength and metabolic rate and maintain metabolically active tissue in older adults (Campbell et al. 1994). Moreover, resistance training has been shown to lower visceral fat, the fat associated with a higher risk of heart disease (Treuth, Hunter, and Kekes-Szabo 1995).

Activity and Diet

When you combine exercise and diet, you can eat more and still achieve a weight loss of 2 pounds (about 1 kilogram) per week:

1,000 calories per day × 7 days = 7,000 calories divided by 3,500 calories per pound = 2 pounds

Exercise tones muscles, improves your appearance, conserves protein, and increases the utilization of fat. The combination of exercise and sensible caloric intake should be a way of life. Let's see how diet and exercise can be combined in a program of weight loss and weight control.

John is 20 pounds (9 kilograms) overweight and in the poor fitness category. He achieves energy balance when his caloric intake equals his typical daily expenditure, 2,500 calories. How should he proceed? John should reduce his caloric intake by 500 calories per day and begin exercising (see table 13.2).

Table 13.2 Sample Weight-Loss Program

20 lb × 3,500 cal/lb = 70,000 cal overweight		Cal	Total cal
Weeks 1 & 2	Exercise = 200 cal/day × 7 days =	1,400	
	Diet = 500 cal/day × 14 days =	7,000	
		8,400	8,400
Weeks 3 & 4	Exercise = 250 cal/day × 14 days =	3,500	
	Diet = 500 cal/day × 14 days =	7,000	
		10,500	18,900
Weeks 5 & 6	Exercise = 300 cal/day × 14 days =	4,200	
	Diet = 500 cal/day × 14 days =	7,000	
		11,200	30,100
Weeks 7 & 8	Exercise = 350 cal/day × 14 days =	4,900	
	Diet = 500 cal/day × 14 days =	7,000	
		11,900	42,000
Weeks 9 & 10	Exercise = 400 cal/day × 14 days =	5,600	
	Diet = 500 cal/day × 14 days =	7,000	
		12,600	54,600
Weeks 11 & 12	Exercise = 450 cal/day × 14 days =	6,300	
	Diet = 500 cal/day × 14 days =	7,000	
		13,300	67,900

After 12 weeks = 67,900 cal lost.

Weeks 13 & 14—forget the diet. Exercise just 150 cal/day (14 days × 150 cal = 2,100 cal). 67,900 + 2,100 = 70,000 cal, or 20 lb.

Now that he has achieved his goal, John has several choices:

• Continue to exercise and eat as he pleases

• Continue activity and a reduced-fat diet

• Return to sedentary habits and restrict caloric intake . . . for life

• Return to sedentary habits and a high-fat diet and regain all the weight he has lost . . . and more

If he chooses to remain active (400 calories of activity daily), he will be able to eat the foods he enjoys and to splurge occasionally on extravagant foods. He should still consider a reduction of fat in the diet, but it is possible that with sufficient activity (e.g., running 4 to 5 miles [6 to 8 kilometers] daily), he will be able to eat whatever he wishes with no adverse effect on his weight or health. However, only a blood lipid profile (cholesterol, LDL, and HDL cholesterol, and triglycerides) will confirm that possibility.

Summary

In the words of a leading obesity researcher, "Exercise is clearly beneficial as a means of losing weight and keeping it off. Given recent studies showing its association with maintenance, it would be difficult to argue that any factor is more important than exercise" (Brownell 1995, p. 124).

Activity is the positive way to achieve weight control without the loss of lean tissue. Dieting is a negative approach that uses deprivation to achieve results. It is not surprising that dieting by itself is seldom successful in the long run. Most weight-loss diets end in failure, with more weight and fat than before the dieting began. Activities such as walking, jogging, or cycling may seem like slow ways to lose weight, but they work. If your activity burns 250 extra calories each day, you'll burn more than 1,500 calories a week. In the course of a year you'll lose more than 20 pounds (9 kilograms). Calories do count, and you should learn how to count them. Turn to chapter 14 for a sensible and effective approach to achieve energy balance and take the first step in your lifelong quest for a trim, healthy body.

ignored. Coaches who encourage such procedures should be held responsible for conducting weight-loss programs when the athlete's season or career is over.

As with weight loss, the weight-gain program includes exercise, diet, and behavior therapy.

- **Exercise:** Includes a strength-training program to build lean body weight and a *reduction* in calorie-burning activities (aerobic exercise, sports) to allow a positive caloric balance.
- **Diet:** Includes an overall increase in calories, with 750 extra calories on strength-training days and 250 extra on nontraining days. The extra calories should be largely from low-fat, protein-rich foods (lean meats, low-fat dairy products, soy protein). A low-fat protein supplement can be used to provide an extra 20 grams (86 calories) of protein daily.
- **Behavior therapy:** If needed, develop a reinforcement schedule to reward gains in lean body weight. Determine a desirable weight, and make steady progress toward that goal.

This program should lead to a gain of about one pound of weight each week. If you attempt to gain weight too fast, much of the gain will be fat. So determine current eating behaviors and plan needed modifications (e.g., more meals, nutritious snacks). Start strength training and watch the scale go up. And remember, return to aerobic exercise and weight control when you achieve the desired body weight.

Health Clubs and Diet Centers

Do health clubs and diet centers figure in your weight-control program? Though both have experienced considerable growth in recent years, you should be cautious in your approach to their services. It may surprise you to learn that neither clubs nor centers are governed by state or local laws. No professional competence or qualifications are required. Hairdressers need a state license, but in most states anyone can open and operate a health club or diet center. Here are some suggestions to help you become a discriminating consumer.

Health Clubs

To help you differentiate a good club from a bad one—an effective program and qualified staff from a fly-by-night organization—you should do the following: Visit the club for a tour and free introductory session. Is the facility clean and well equipped? Does the equipment meet your needs? Are patrons satisfied; do they encourage you to join? Ask about the staff's qualifications and credentials. Do they have degrees in the field from reputable institutions? Do they have experience? Are they certified? Are they all trained in emergency response? The American College of Sports Medicine (ACSM) certifies health and fitness instructors and program directors who meet educational and experience standards and successfully complete a rigorous test. ACSM publishes standards for health clubs and has a brochure to help you evaluate a health club. Write to ACSM at P.O. Box 1440, Indianapolis, IN 46206-1440, or visit their Web site (**www.acsm.org**) to request the brochure or other services.

When you decide to join a club, avoid long-term contracts. Be wary of discounts and other high-pressure come-ons; they may be signs of a failing business or high member turnover. Sign up for a few months or until you are absolutely certain that the club meets your needs. Then become active in a member advisory group that works with management to maintain and upgrade staff qualifications, facilities, and equipment.

Diet Centers

Although diet centers provide dieting advice and encouragement, few boast the services of a registered dietitian, and fewer still have an on-site medical director. Most centers sell expensive vitamins, diet foods, and other products to their clients. Some clients lose weight, often at a rapid rate, indicating significant loss of water and lean tissue. Some centers advise against exercise, because clients following their program are often too listless to participate.

If you or a friend are considering the services of a diet center, follow the advice I provided regarding health clubs. Visit, ask questions, and by all means ask about qualifications. Is a registered dietitian on the staff? Is a reputable local physician associated with the center? Most important, ask about the program's long-term success rate. Then ask to contact some of the diet center's clients. Ask yourself if the center provides any service you cannot provide for yourself. The existence of so many centers suggests that the simple facts of energy balance and weight control have reached too few, that individuals lack the information, opportunity, or will to take control of their eating and activity behaviors.

Weight-Control Fallacies

Let's review some of the fallacies associated with weight loss.

Lose Inches, Not Pounds

This is the "come-on" of the figure salon, where they try to appeal to people who don't want to work hard enough to achieve real fat and weight loss. Of course, it is possible to improve one's appearance with exercises that merely tone muscles and improve posture. The fallacy is that while you are shaping the body, you are ignoring the engine, rusty hoses, and other parts (i.e., the heart and blood vessels) and missing out on the health benefits associated with body weight and fat loss. Typically the inches are not lost at all; a slightly tighter pull on the measuring tape gives the impression of progress. Fitness and health, like beauty, are more than skin deep.

Spot Reduction

There is very limited evidence that fat can be removed from specific areas (spots) by localized exercises. One study showed a mere one millimeter of spot reduction after six weeks of exercise. Avid tennis players have about the same skinfold on both arms, even though one arm is larger and more muscular.

Dunlop's Disease

My friend Ted once tried sit-ups to get rid of "Dunlop's Disease," where his tummy "done lopped" over his belt. He worked up to 400 sit-ups daily with no success. I showed him a study conducted by Dr. Frank Katch and colleagues at the University of Massachusetts. They collected fat biopsies from several sites before and after a four-week training program consisting entirely of sit-ups. Posttraining analysis of fat cells revealed that the fat came from all the fat storage areas measured, not just abdominal fat (McArdle, Katch, and Katch 1994). What about Ted? He became an ultramarathoner, training for and running 100-mile (161-kilometer) races, and his tummy ceased to be a problem. The moral of this story is burn off sufficient calories, and the spots and inches will take care of themselves.

Exercise Devices

You've seen the advertisements for passive exercise: electrical stimulation, vibrating machines, sauna shorts, and body wraps, devices that promise weight or fat loss without effort on your part. Sorry, they just don't work. Passive devices don't burn enough calories, electrical stimulation is not equivalent to voluntary exercise, vibrating devices do not break up fat and wash it away in the circulation, and tight pants or wraps do not remove fat with heat and massage. Spend the same amount of time in moderate exercise and you will get results, including the health benefits you miss with passive exercise.

The advertising usually claims that with a few minutes of "almost effortless" activity you will get a firm, healthy, athletic body. They use attractive models, celebrities, or pro athletes to tout the product, and there is usually a big discount if you act immediately. If you are uncertain, ask your physician or local health club professional (certified by the American College of Sports Medicine) for advice. My advice: try the product before you buy. Don't sign a long-term contract for any type of exercise program or device. And remember, a brisk walk burns more calories than most passive devices, and it's a lot more fun.

Drugs and Surgery

Laxatives and diuretics remove only water (dehydration). Amphetamines are sometimes prescribed to suppress the appetite, a dangerous approach to lifelong weight control. Reputable physicians prescribe anorectic agents (appetite suppressants) as part of a total program with diet, exercise, and behavior therapy. But they need to avoid increasing doses and the risk of dependency. Recently a weight-control drug combination was associated with development of heart valve problems. And weight-control drugs, when they work, have to be taken forever to achieve long-term weight control. Research on the genetic component of obesity may lead to future therapies, but that will never remove the need to balance caloric intake and expenditure.

Lipectomy and liposuction are surgical techniques used to remove unwanted fat. Though lipectomy certainly removes fat and reduces weight, some studies suggest the fat may be regenerated, especially if caloric intake continues to exceed expenditure. Liposuction, which involves vacuuming of fat cells from abdominal, thigh, and other deposits, is generally safe, but no surgery is without risk. And there is no proof that surgical removal of superficial fat will change heart disease or other risk factors, unless it is accompanied with diet and exercise. Other forms of surgery are reserved for cases of morbid obesity, defined as more than 100 pounds (45 kilograms) overweight. One operation involves bypass of a portion of the small intestine, whereas a less complicated approach uses staples to fashion a smaller stomach. Obviously, surgery is an expensive and potentially dangerous approach to weight control.

Eating Disorders

The most tragic fallacy is the adoption of dangerous eating behaviors in an effort to achieve an unattainable ideal: a slim, trim figure. When being thin becomes an obsession, when self-worth becomes associated with slimness, the stage is set for eating disorders. *Bulimia* is a disorder characterized by a binge/purge cycle. Those with mild cases purge (vomit) occasionally to avoid weight gain, while those with more serious cases combine binge/purge with laxatives or diuretics, risking serious metabolic and psychological problems.

Anorexia nervosa is a serious psychological problem characterized by a distorted body image and a refusal to eat. Sometimes the behavior is associated with drugs or with obsessive exercise. If not treated, the individual may experience serious medical complications, including death as starvation compromises the heart and other organs. Eating disorders are more common among young women who seek to please others, who try to be perfect. Fortunately, psychological therapy and medical treatments are available to victims who seek help.

Smoking?

It is sad to see young women smoking cigarettes, but it is tragic to hear that they continue the habit to avoid weight gain. Though it is true that smokers gain some weight when they quit, the amount is not so excessive that it can't be eliminated with diet and exercise. Moreover, the health consequences of smoking far outweigh the effect of any weight gain. Develop an addiction to exercise to replace the addiction to nicotine.

To avoid contributing to the development of eating disorders, don't nag teenagers about weight problems. Minimize the emphasis on body weight, girth, and fat values and focus on how they feel and function.

Schedule family activities followed by sensible family meals. Use desserts sparingly, and stock fruits instead of high-fat or high-sugar snacks. Be aware of eating behaviors and seek help early if eating disorders arise.

Summary

This chapter has presented ways to use activity, dieting, and behavioral therapy in your lifelong effort to achieve energy balance and weight control. In years past young folks were more active and had more metabolically active tissue, so weight control wasn't a big problem. With inactivity and poor food choices, overweight and obesity are epidemic. With age and responsibilities come even less activity and a further decline in metabolically active tissue, including muscle. Eventually, winter weight gains fail to melt off in the spring, and energy balance becomes a major issue. I've reached the stage of life where I must exercise more or eat less if I want to maintain my body weight, cholesterol, waist size, and self-respect. Because I already engage in a considerable amount of exercise and have already reduced the fat in my diet, I am faced with the unhappy prospect of life with fewer calories. But don't feel sorry for me. I've come this far enjoying an enormous appetite and a great love of food, and it is time that I learn some self-control. Guess I'll have to review the section on behavior therapy.

PART V

Performance in Work and Sport

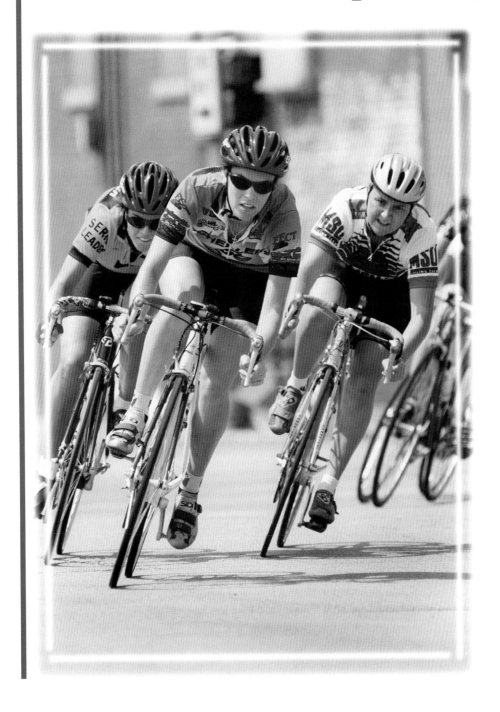

On a typical day, most of us spend about eight hours in sleep and eight hours at work. The rest is largely dedicated to preparation for one or the other, or for so-called leisure-time pursuits, including activity and sport. Improve fitness to enhance work capacity or performance in sport, and the sleep will take care of itself.

Beyond health, even beyond fitness, there is the desire to perform at a high level, to achieve one's potential. To do this one must set goals, then design and carry out a systematic plan to achieve them. The final step is to achieve what you trained for, sometimes in a public performance or event. We usually think of performing in sports, races, or other competitions, but some people train for cross-country bicycle trips, mountain climbs, or other private personal goals. Far too few train to improve their work capacity, to be industrial athletes capable of impressive performances in the workplace.

This section will help you improve your performance in work and sport. I'll show you how to use simple psychological skills to help you perform better, to play your best game more often. And I'll discuss how to prepare for and perform in a variety of terrestrial environments, including heat, cold, and altitude.

15

Performance at Work

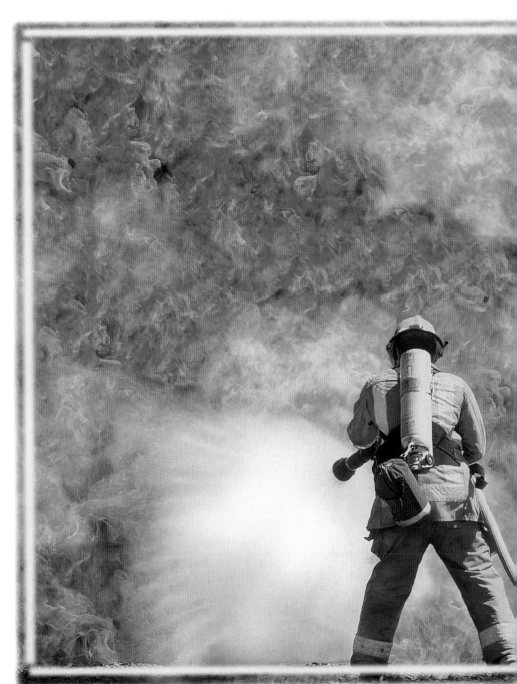

"In order that people may be happy in their work, these three things are needed: They must be fit for it. They must not do too much of it. And they must have a sense of success in it."

John Ruskin

Until recently, the primary source of power for the production of useful work was derived from the contractions of muscles, both human and animal. Of course, people devised ways to augment muscle power with the ingenious use of wind and water, but it was not until the 18th century that mechanization began to reduce the need for muscular work. Machines were devised to supplement or replace human effort. Robots, computers, and other devices have replaced the need for human muscle power. Today, when men and women go to work, few are required to engage in arduous muscular effort.

Much of the credit for the reduction in physical labor must go to the inventors and engineers whose attempts at mechanization and, more recently, computers and robotics have made work relatively effortless. Some credit also is due to specialists in ergonomics, the scientific study of work. Work physiologists, psychologists, and engineers combine to study men and women in their working environment, with the goal of adapting the job to the ability of the average worker. At the same time, labor-saving devices have eliminated the need for muscular work at home, and the automobile makes the task of getting to and from work physically effortless.

The consequences of these trends are obvious: The average worker is incapable of delivering a full day's effort in a physically demanding job, and degenerative diseases associated with inactivity, such as heart disease—the nation's number one killer—are epidemic. If job requirements are continually lowered to meet the ability of the average unfit and overweight worker, the trend will continue. Perhaps it is time for a change; perhaps we could benefit by working up to job requirements, not down. Perhaps it is time to adapt the worker to the job rather than just adapting the job to the worker.

■ This chapter will help you

- understand the relationship between fitness and work capacity, and see why fitness is good for business;
- improve work performance and job satisfaction and appreciate the importance of physical maintenance to performance and satisfaction; and
- better integrate your job and your lifestyle.

Fitness and Work

Certain jobs still require strength and endurance at least some of the time. Workers in heavy industry, construction, agriculture, forestry, public safety, and the military are often required to engage in strenuous effort. Without proper conditioning, the stress of arduous work can be unpleasant or worse, so concern for these employees' health and safety has prompted screening procedures to make sure the worker is capable of meeting job demands. Many companies have instituted employee fitness programs to help workers meet and maintain required levels of work capacity.

Experience shows that unfit workers can become a safety hazard to themselves as well as to co-workers. Fit workers are more productive than their sedentary colleagues, are absent fewer days, and are far less likely to incur job-related disabilities or retire early due to heart or other degenerative diseases. Moreover,

solution to the overwhelming weekend congestion on highways, beaches, tennis courts, golf courses, and ski lifts and even in wilderness areas. The four-day (10 hours per day) workweek has been tried with considerable success in a number of industries. Schedules can be staggered to provide flexible three-day rest periods. Some possible workweeks are M-T-W-Th, T-W-Th-F, W-Th-F-Sa, even Su-M-T-W. Some people may even prefer to take their "weekend" during the week (F-Sa-Su-M). When combined with flextime, the four-day workweek can further humanize the world of work, thereby providing a greater opportunity for a creative adaptation to life.

Home Office

Perhaps the most appealing alternative to the traditional workweek is telecommuting from your home office. Even if this is done only one or two days each week, it saves money, time, and frayed nerves and allows a more flexible approach for a young or single parent. The time usually spent commuting can be spent at work, freeing other time for family and individual activities, including food preparation and exercise. Money saved on transportation and clothing costs can be used to enhance the quality of life. I belong to an organization that once spent thousands to bring officers and committees to the city of its headquarters for meetings. Today we accomplish most of our business via teleconference. Soon we'll be able to sit at home and use the computer to meet, share documents, and balance budgets, face to face. Though the home office will never replace the need for in-person communication, it does provide another way to free the employee from rigid, outdated workplace requirements, and it opens the door to the active life.

Occupational Physiology

Physiology, the study of the human body, is becoming increasingly important in the workplace to determine job demands and aid in the selection of workers; to work-harden, train, and cross-train workers to improve performance and reduce injuries; to rehabilitate injured workers; and to confront job discrimination according to age, gender, race, or disability. This section considers some of the current issues and provides a fair approach to hiring.

Fit to Work

Finding the right person for the job can often be difficult. Employers use high school and college transcripts, written tests, letters of recommendation, background checks, even psychological and drug tests to try to find good employees. When the job demands physical performance, many employers are turning to job-related tests to aid the selection process.

Job-Related Tests

Job-related tests have replaced old-fashioned fitness tests in the workplace. Development of a valid test of work capacity begins with a job task analysis to select important work tasks. The candidate test is then administered to successful employees to ensure its usefulness and to select a cutoff score. Thereafter, the test can be used to select new employees, to ensure that current employees maintain work capacity, and as a return-to-work evaluation following injury or illness.

Job Demands

Dr. Paul Davis has developed a job-related test for municipal (structural) firefighters. The test incorporates actual elements of the job, including carrying hoses up several flights of stairs, a chopping task, pulling a heavy hose, and a victim carry. Though some people may argue with the cutoff score used by a particular department, few would say that the test fails to represent the demands of the job. Many departments use this or a similar test to select among the many candidates for the job. Unfortunately, only a few departments demand that their firefighters pass the test annually (Dotson, Santa Maria, and Davis 1976). Dr. Davis' studies show that the fitness and health of public service personnel (police, fire) decline at about the same rate as the sedentary, overweight population. Their heart disease rates are the same as the sedentary population. Taxpayers pay for their failure to practice healthy habits and maintain fitness and health.

Ergonomics

For decades the goal of ergonomics has been to adapt the job to the worker. Scientists and engineers have attempted to ease the burden on the worker by making adjustments in tools or work processes. When conditions or costs limit these adjustments, it makes sense to adapt workers to the job. When the job is demanding, the best approach is to select individuals physically suited for the work and to maintain their work capacity with an ongoing job-related fitness program. Some companies have begun to view their workers as highly trained industrial athletes. They recruit, train, maintain, and cross-train those with the physical capacity to do the work.

Physical Maintenance

Job-related testing accomplishes little if it is only used on recruits. The only way to maintain physical work capacity throughout a worker's career is to require annual testing and participation in a job-related fitness program. Fire departments are known for the care they give their equipment. They purchase rigorously tested equipment and maintain it with meticulous upkeep. Yet they will hire employees who barely pass a selection test and then ignore the need for ongoing physical maintenance. Unfortunately, the need to maintain work capacity has become a pawn in the collective bargaining process.

A well-designed program maintains or builds the aerobic and muscular capabilities needed on the job while meeting the employees' health and wellness needs. The program also addresses injury prevention with stretching and strengthening exercises, insures needed heat or altitude acclimatization, and teaches the importance of nutrition and hydration. When job-related fitness is a high priority, work time is provided to maintain job performance. This is good business in that fit workers are less likely to sustain disabling injuries and are quicker to return to work after injury. Fitness improves performance in the heat, shortens the time required for acclimatization, and dramatically raises work output. In our studies of wildland firefighters, highly fit and motivated workers regularly outperform less-fit workers by a factor of three to one (Sharkey 1981)!

Equal Opportunity

A major feature of the workplace during the past 30 years has been the effort to provide equal employment opportunities. A series of federal laws has attempted to eliminate discrimination based on age, gender, race, or disability.

Age

The Age Discrimination in Employment Act (ADEA) of 1967 outlawed job discrimination based on age, except when age was a bona fide occupational qualification (BFOQ). The BFOQ requires that the effects of advancing age make it impossible for all or most individuals above a certain age to do a job, or it is impossible to assess work capacity with a job-related test, or both. Neither condition of the BFOQ is defensible. For years, Congress exempted fire and law-enforcement personnel from the ADEA, assuming that age was a BFOQ. However, a large study commissioned by the Equal Employment Opportunity Commission (EEOC) found that age was poorly correlated with performance, and that job-related tests accurately reflected work capacity (Landy 1992).

Studies of fire and law-enforcement personnel indicated the dismal level of physical readiness of emergency service personnel. Fitness declines rapidly in this sedentary population, and body fat levels double during the 20-year career (Davis and Starck 1980). With this physical decline comes a high rate of heart disease, which, surprisingly, is viewed as a job-related disability. Taxpayers deserve the best public servants available, and age alone does not insure career-long fitness for duty. The solution is to test recruits and follow up with annual performance evaluations, coupled with a job-related physical maintenance (fitness) program. Unfortunately, in spite of the studies, Congress has voted to reinstate the exemption to the ADEA!

Too Old?

Management considered George too old to become a "smoke jumper," but not too old to conduct the physical training program for this elite bunch of firefighters. The jumpers are wildland firefighters who parachute into the wilderness to battle wildfires. When the fire is contained, they load up their gear, all 125 pounds (56.7 kilograms) of it, and "pack it out" several miles to the nearest trailhead. As he approached retirement from his university teaching position, George took advantage of the ADEA and signed up for jumper training. At the tender age of 58 he passed the arduous physical tests, jump training, and field tests such as the pack-out, and he became a smoke jumper. Age alone says little about performance or the size of a person's heart.

Gender

In the 1970s, with the help of the Civil Rights Act of 1964, women began to seek employment in previously male-dominated jobs such as firefighting, law enforcement, construction, and the military. In many cases the transition took place with little fanfare, but in some it has been a struggle. Men still question women's ability to carry out jobs that require considerable upper-body strength. Job-related tests used to select employees have been labeled discriminatory when they disqualify

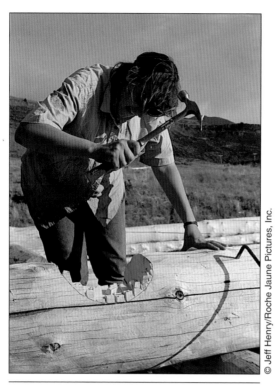

Women have worked to achieve success in formerly male-dominated occupations.

© Jeff Henry/Roche Jaune Pictures, Inc.

a large proportion of women. For example, in a test of more than 6,000 recruits for the Chicago Fire Department, no women scored in the top 2,000. Because there were fewer than 200 openings, the test appeared to discriminate against women.

The Federal Uniform Guidelines for Employee Selection Procedures (EEOC 1978) state that a selection test has adverse impact when a class of employees scores less than 80 percent (four-fifths) of the rate of the highest class. Therefore, when women pass at a rate that is less than 80 percent of the men's pass rate, the employer is required to demonstrate the validity of the test and why it is necessary. When job tasks require upper-body strength it is virtually impossible to avoid adverse impact, because women average 50 to 60 percent of men's upper-body strength.

Unfortunately, many valid tests have been discontinued for fear of adverse impact and lawsuits brought by individuals as well as state and federal human rights and equal opportunity commissions. In my view, this is a disservice to women. Performance in sport proves that women are capable of training to meet physical challenges. Women's world records in running are just 10 percent below those of men in distances ranging from 100 meters to the marathon (42 kilometers, or 26 miles, 385 yards). My experience with the women of the U.S. cross-country ski team and with wildland firefighters has convinced me that many women have what it takes to succeed in difficult occupations. Women athletes train to build muscle strength and endurance, and women can train to compete in formerly male-only jobs.

Tara's Story

Tara was a graduate student in exercise science and my research assistant when she decided to become a smoke jumper. At that time only a few women had made it through training to become jumpers. Tara was an endurance athlete who weighed barely enough to qualify for training, so she designed and carried out a weight-training program to gain strength and lean body weight. After several months of serious training she successfully completed the entrance test and training, including the pack-out—a 3-mile (4.8-kilometer) hike with a 110-pound (50-kilogram) pack (equal to her lean body weight). This determined lady would not be satisfied with watered-down qualifications. She wanted to be accepted on her merits as a qualified worker, not a token woman or an affirmative-action hire.

Until women are given the chance to work up to defensible job standards, we'll never know how good they can be. Establish valid job-related tests, advertise the standards, and provide preemployment training programs. If few women qualify, don't panic and lower the standards. Hold firm, and watch as women come forth to accept the challenge.

Racial/Ethnic Groups

Studies in work physiology do not suggest racial or ethnic differences in work capacity. With some people doubting the validity of race as a useful classification and others downplaying the existence of meaningful racial differences, there is little justification for a lengthy discussion. What is clear is that job-related work-capacity tests do not unfairly impact racial or ethnic groups. Indeed, valid work-capacity tests can be considered color-blind.

People With Disabilities

The Americans with Disabilities Act (ADA) of 1991 was enacted to insure employment opportunities and reasonable accommodations for persons with disabilities. The act also mandates improved access for those with disabilities. The ADA endorses the use of valid preemployment tests as an objective way to determine a person's ability to do the job. It allows postemployment medical examinations so long as all workers are included and the results remain confidential. And the act encourages employers to make reasonable accommodations for persons with disabilities.

Summary

Performance in physically demanding work is related to fitness; the harder the work, the higher the relationship to measures of aerobic and muscular fitness. Therefore, when selecting employees for hard work it makes good sense to use a job-related work-capacity test to hire those most suited for the work. But selection isn't enough: An ongoing job-related fitness or physical maintenance program is necessary to make certain that employees maintain the capacity to do the job. The ideal plan involves a job-related selection test, a well-designed fitness program to maintain work capacity, an employee health/wellness program for health, and annual retesting with the work-capacity test. When combined with ergonomics, safety, and injury prevention, you have a comprehensive approach to employee health, safety, and performance.

A final note to extol an additional workplace benefit for those who pursue the active life. Studies in the United States and Canada indicate a positive relationship between leisure-time physical activity and personal income; as the level of activity increases, so does the level of income. Now everyone with a college education knows that a correlation does not imply cause and effect, so it doesn't mean that you'll make more money if you become more active. Frequently a relationship can be explained by the fact that behaviors are interrelated, that two are related to a third variable. Indeed, there is a well-known relationship between education level and income—income rises with education. And there is a positive relationship between education and level of activity, and that helps to explain why activity is related to income (Stephens, Jacobs, and White 1985).

It's no secret that vigorous, enthusiastic individuals are more likely to be hired. Once hired, raises and promotions should be based primarily on performance. Because activity and fitness improve health, performance, morale, and safety, it seems reasonable that vigorous and enthusiastic workers will be retained, rewarded, and promoted to more responsible positions. In this era of corporate downsizing and layoffs, it seems prudent to do all you can to acquire, retain, and enhance opportunities for challenging and personally rewarding employment. Don't ignore the role of activity and fitness in the workplace.

16

Performance in Sport

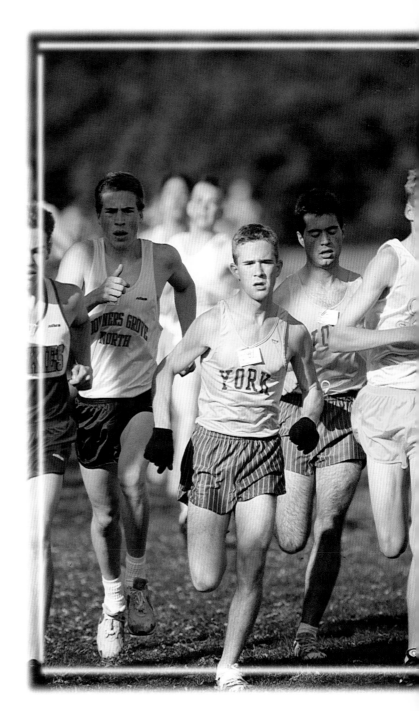

"Don't play sports to get in shape; get in shape to play sports!"

Anonymous

319

In this chapter, I tell you how to prepare for athletic competition safely and effectively so that you can enjoy the intense pleasure and excitement of sport and competition, without the risk of fatigue, overtraining, injury, or illness. Opportunities for adult (masters, senior, veteran) competition include road races, orienteering, track and field, swimming, alpine and cross-country skiing, tennis, racquetball, handball, golf, softball, volleyball, bowling, judo, karate, and many others. Adults participate according to age group, and it is not unusual to find active athletes of 60, 70, and even 80 years of age. A few continue to participate in races beyond their 100th birthdays, as did the late Larry Lewis, an indefatigable runner and a waiter at a posh San Francisco hotel. If you like to train and enjoy the thrill of competition, of getting high on your own hormones, this section is for you. But remember, you must train before you compete.

■ This chapter will help you

- utilize the principles of training,
- improve performance in your favorite sport,
- use diet to enhance performance, and
- develop psychological skills to help you play your best game more often.

Principles of Training

This section introduces 12 important physiological principles (adapted from Sharkey 1986) that you should follow to make steady progress in your training and to avoid illness and injury.

Principle 1: Readiness

The value of training depends on the physiological and psychological readiness of the individual. Because readiness comes with maturation, physically immature (prepubertal) individuals lack the physiological preparedness to respond completely to training. Readiness also implies the need for adequate nutrition and rest to benefit from training. Psychological readiness refers to the commitment to delay gratification and make the sacrifices involved in sustained training.

Principle 2: Adaptation

Training induces subtle changes as the body adapts to the added demands. Dr. Ned Fredrick, a friend and a noted sport scientist, calls training for sport a gentle pastime in which we coax subtle changes from the body. The day-to-day changes are so small as to be unmeasurable; weeks and even months of patient progress are required to achieve measurable adaptations. Try to rush the process, and you risk illness, injury, or both.

Typical adaptations include

- increased enzyme proteins or contractile proteins;
- improved respiration, heart function, circulation, and blood volume;
- improved muscular endurance, strength, or power; and
- tougher bones, ligaments, tendons, and connective tissue.

gospel of fitness and health to the lay public. His YMCA workshops were legendary for the enormous energy exhibited by this traveling prophet of fitness. He was so busy he had little time for himself.

Sometime after his retirement he returned to the pool, site of youthful success in competitive swimming. Before long he was setting national and then world records in his age group. I'll never forget his contributions or his delight at finding athletic success in his eighth decade. It's never too late to start, or to start over.

Training Fallacies

You may hear about some other so-called "principles of training"; you should be aware that some of them are actually fallacies or misconceptions. These often-quoted principles are not true and have no basis in medical or scientific research.

Fallacy 1: No Pain, No Gain

Although serious training is often difficult and sometimes unpleasant, it shouldn't hurt. In fact, well-prepared athletes can perform difficult events in a state of euphoria, free of pain and oblivious to discomfort. Marathon winners sometimes seem to finish full of vitality, whereas others appear near collapse. Pain is not a natural consequence of exercise or training; it is a sign of a problem that shouldn't be ignored. During exercise the body produces natural opiates, called endorphins, that can mask discomfort of the effort. If you experience real pain during training, you should back off. If the pain persists, have the problem evaluated.

Discomfort, on the other hand, can accompany difficult aspects of training such as heavy lifting, intense interval training, or long-distance effort. Discomfort is a natural consequence of the lactic acid that accompanies the anaerobic effort of lifting or intervals, or of the muscle fatigue, microscopic muscle damage (microtrauma), and soreness that come with long-distance training. I would accept this statement: No discomfort, no excellence. Overload sometimes requires working at the upper limit of strength, intensity, or endurance, and that can be temporarily uncomfortable. If exercise results in pain, it is probably excessive. The next two fallacies are also associated with the "no pain, no gain" misconception.

Fallacy 2: You Must Break Down Muscle to Improve

Microtrauma sometimes occurs in muscle during vigorous training and competition, but it isn't a necessary or even a desirable outcome of training. Runners have shown significant microtrauma at the end of a marathon with long downhill stretches that require eccentric muscular contractions (contractions of a lengthening muscle). Eccentric contractions are a major cause of muscle soreness, which is associated with muscle trauma, reduced force output, and a prolonged (four to six weeks) period of recovery. Excessive trauma doesn't help training; it stops it.

Weight lifters can traumatize muscle with excess weight or repetitions, but that is not a necessary stage in the development of strength. Neither pain nor injury is a normal consequence of training, and you should avoid both.

Fallacy 3: Go for the Burn

This popular statement is often heard among bodybuilders who do numerous repetitions and sets to build, shape, and define muscles. The burn they describe is probably due to the increased acidity associated with elevated levels of lactic acid in the muscle. Although this sensation isn't dangerous, it isn't a necessary part of a strength program designed to improve performance.

Fallacy 4: Lactic Acid Causes Muscle Soreness

This fallacy has been around for years, without any basis in fact. Although lactic acid may be produced in contractions that lead to soreness, the lactic acid isn't the cause of the soreness. Lactic acid is cleared from muscle and blood within an hour of the exercise. Soreness comes 24 hours or more after the effort, long after the lactic acid has been removed or metabolized. Soreness follows unfamiliar exertion or a long layoff and is probably associated with microtrauma to muscle and connective tissue and the swelling that results. After recovery, additional exposure to the activity will yield less soreness.

Fallacy 5: Muscle Turns to Fat (or Vice Versa)

Another common misconception is that when an athlete stops training, muscle can turn to fat. Muscle will no more turn to fat than fat will turn to muscle. Both are highly specialized tissues with specific functions. Muscles are composed of long, spaghettilike fibers with contractile proteins designed to exert force. Fat cells are round receptacles designed to store fat. Training increases the size of muscle fibers (hypertrophy), and detraining reduces their size (atrophy). Excess caloric consumption causes fat cells to grow in size as they store more fat. The cells shrink when you burn more calories than you eat. But long, thin muscle fibers do not change into spherical blobs of fat, or vice versa.

Fallacy 6: I Ran Out of Wind

Athletes often have the sensation of running out of wind when they run too fast for their level of training. The sensation comes from the lungs and reflects another discomfort of exertion. However, it is more likely to be due to an excess of carbon dioxide than a lack of oxygen or air. Carbon dioxide is produced during the oxidative metabolism of carbohydrate, and it is the primary stimulus for respiration. So, when carbon dioxide levels are high, as they are during vigorous effort, they cause distress signals in the lungs. The respiratory system thinks it is more important to rid the body of excess CO_2 than it is to bring in more O_2. Excess CO_2 is a sign that you have exceeded your lactate threshold, that you are working above your level of training. Become familiar with the sensation and what it is telling you; ignore it, and you will soon become exhausted.

The Physiology of Training

The physiology of training, which studies the response of the body to training, has received a great deal of attention in recent years. Working together, coaches, athletes, and sports scientists have contributed to a growing body of knowledge about how the body responds to the demands of systematic training. This section provides an overview of training to guide the development and conduct of your program.

Energy Training

To tailor a training program suited to your needs, you first must know the energy sources required in the activity. Figure 16.1 illustrates the relative contribution of anaerobic and aerobic energy sources in relation to the distance or duration of running events (use the time scale to estimate energy sources for other activities). Next, it helps to know something about your individual capabilities, both anaerobic and aerobic. If you are eager to prepare for a marathon, for which the energy source is primarily aerobic, you should be as strong as possible in aerobic fitness. If your event is primarily anaerobic, like a 100-meter swim, you will need anaerobic capabilities, along with the aerobic capacity to support training and enhance recovery. Once you know the energy sources used in the activity and your own capabilities, you can begin to design your training program.

To tailor a training program suited to your needs, you first must know the energy sources required in the activity.

Year-Round Training

Though it is possible to make significant improvements in aerobic energy sources in as little as two to three months, a year-round program is bound to be safer and more effective (see figure 16.2). All training begins with an aerobic buildup, a period of slow distance work that builds stamina and neuromuscular efficiency.

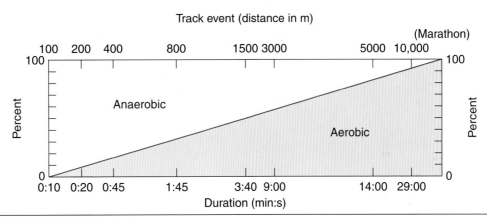

Figure 16.1 Anaerobic and aerobic energy sources in relation to distance and duration of events. Shorter events are primarily anaerobic. For distances greater than 1,500 meters (longer than four minutes), training should concentrate on aerobic fitness.

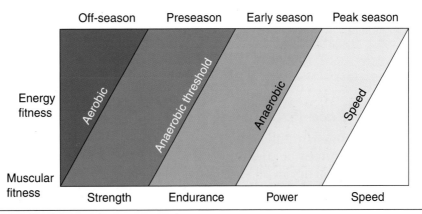

Figure 16.2 Seasonal training goals.

Table 16.1 Seasonal Training Goals and Methods

Season	Training goals	Training methods
Off-season	Aerobic fitness of slow-twitch fibers	Long, slow distance, medium distance, Fartlek,* hills
Preseason	Raise anaerobic threshold and aerobic fitness of fast oxidative glycolytic (FOG) fibers	Long intervals (2-5 min), Fartlek, pace work, fast distance
Early season	Anaerobic capability and short-term energy and speed	Medium intervals (60-90 s), short intervals (30-60 s), sprints
Peak season	Maintain training gains and achieve peak performances	Reduce training volume, emphasize quality not quantity

*Fartlek—a medium-distance effort that consists of faster sections followed by slower ones for recovery.

Once a sound aerobic foundation has been established, you are ready to train the upper end of your aerobic capability, the lactate threshold. This is accomplished by interval training, using long intervals (two to five minutes). Anaerobic training then follows with shorter and faster efforts (30 to 90 seconds). Finally, and only if speed is required in the event, sprints can be added to the program (table 16.1).

The year-round approach to training provides the strong foundation needed to compete successfully. It minimizes the risk of injury that accompanies anaerobic and speed training. It leads to a competitive peak that can be sustained for a month or more and provides for a postseason recovery period prior to a renewed training effort. If you are involved in several activities and cannot devote 12 months to any one, use the same approach but shorten each phase. Always allow at least 1 month each for aerobic and anaerobic threshold buildups. If necessary, use the first few weeks of the competitive season for anaerobic and speed training, but don't expect your best performances until later in the season (Sharkey 1986).

Heart Rate Monitors

Athletes often use heart rate monitors (see figure 16.3) to make sure that they are training at the correct intensity. The best monitors are those that use the electrical signal from the heart (ECG). One popular version transmits the signal from the chest to a wrist monitor that displays the rate and stores heart rates for later analysis. If you decide to use a monitor, you will still need to listen to your body, to become familiar with respiratory and other signs of distress. Use the monitor to estimate your anaerobic threshold, then become aware of your breathing at that level of exertion. You'll need to be able to sense your effort when you get in a race.

Race-Pace Training

To ensure the specificity of training and the development of needed energy sources, be sure to spend part of your time on race-pace training. If your goal is to ski or run a 35-minute 10 kilometer (6.2 miles) course, you'll have to average 3.5 minutes per kilometer. To provide the physiological and psychological base for

Muscular Fitness Training

As sport becomes more competitive at every level, it becomes necessary to invest more time in muscular fitness training. You should evaluate the muscular demands of your sport as well as your strengths and weak points. Then you can proceed to develop a program to improve the strength, muscular endurance, power, or speed you need to reach your goals.

• **Off-season:** This is the time for strength training. Select important muscle groups in the upper body, trunk, and legs and engage in a program following the prescriptions presented in chapter 10. Don't develop more strength than you need. When your strength is adequate for the sport, move on to the next phase of training.

• **Preseason:** By now you should be moving into power and/or muscular endurance training. As the season approaches, make the exercises more sport-specific, more like the movements of the sport. Power is developed in 15 to 25 repetitions maximum (RM) sets done as fast as possible. Short-term (anaerobic) endurance is improved in sets of 15 to 25 RM also, so this phase of muscular fitness training can achieve two goals.

• **Early season:** From now on the emphasis is on speed and the maintenance of gains in strength, endurance, and power. Practice sport skills at high speed to become more comfortable with speed and to improve neuromuscular coordination. Once-a-week maintenance sessions will retain strength and power gains.

How Much Strength?

For endurance sports (e.g., swimming, cross-country skiing), strength in a muscle group is adequate when it exceeds 2.5 times the force used in a typical stroke. Stated another way, the load should not exceed 40 percent of your strength. For example, if you need 20 pounds (9.1 kilograms) of force in the freestyle arm pull, you should have at least 50 pounds, or 22.7 kilograms (20 pounds times 2.5 equals 50 pounds), of strength in the muscle group. Additional strength isn't likely to improve performance.

When I took up cross-country ski racing, I found that my upper body lacked the strength, power, and endurance to maintain vigorous poling throughout a race. So I undertook an off-season strength program to build up the triceps, deltoids, lats, and abdominal muscles used in poling. I did the bench press, dips, and other general exercises for the triceps, along with the more ski-specific modified lat exercise. And I increased the attention usually afforded my abdominal muscles, using weighted sit-ups, the basket hang, and an abdominal machine. In the preseason I switched to more specific exercises, including the rollerboard for power and short-term endurance and extended sessions on roller skis for long-term endurance. The early season included some power training with short sprints, using only poles for propulsion.

What did all this effort yield? Well, my technique and race times improved significantly, as did my enjoyment of the sport (Sharkey 1984). Evaluate the muscular demands of your sport and get started on a program. As you proceed to develop particular muscle groups, don't ignore flexibility, and don't forget to maintain balance by training opposite sides of the joint. Excessive attention to one muscle group, such as the quadriceps on the front of the thigh, could lead to muscle imbalance and a greater risk of injury.

Combining Strength and Endurance Training

Many athletes conduct concurrent strength and aerobic endurance training in the same muscle group, such as the thigh, with squats for strength and cycling for aerobic endurance. Early research suggested that endurance training interfered with the full development of strength (Hickson 1980). A recent study of 45 male and female subjects supports the contention that combined strength and endurance training can suppress some of the adaptations to strength training. Gains in strength were greater with strength-only training. With female subjects the combined training raised the level of the stress hormone cortisol. Surprisingly, the combined training augmented the number of capillaries per muscle fiber, a measure important to endurance (Bell et al. 2000).

If you need high levels of strength, focus on strength training. Evidence exists that experienced athletes are able to thrive in concurrent strength and endurance training. Because concurrent training requires synthesis of strength and endurance proteins, it is important to consume up to 1.8 grams of good-quality protein per kilogram of body weight daily.

In table 16.4 you'll find a format you can use to develop a program for your sport. Figure 16.4 provides a worksheet for program development, and figure 16.5 illustrates a sample program.

Table 16.4   Developing Your Muscular Fitness Program

1. Determine the muscular fitness requirements of the sport or activity.

2. Identify the major muscle groups and movements involved.

3. Select exercises to develop muscular fitness in upper body, trunk, and leg muscles.

4. Make adjustments for strengths and weaknesses.[a]

5. Establish training goals, set up a schedule, and get started. Remember to keep good records and to test progress every few weeks.

For more on training for sports see Sharkey 1986.

[a]Use fewer sets for strong areas, more for those in need of extra help.

The Psychology of Performance

Sport is a study in cooperation and competition. The quality of the overall experience depends on cooperation. Tennis opponents agree to cooperate by calling lines fairly, keeping track of the score, and observing the written rules and etiquette of the game. Fair, enjoyable competition is impossible without a high degree of cooperation. Top competitors often train together. They share training programs, new ideas, aches, pains, even dreams. Even during competition they cooperate, sharing equipment, encouragement, and the experience itself.

Muscular Fitness Program Planner

Sport _____   Position _____

Season _____   Goals _____

Individual strengths _____

Weak points _____

Body Part	Exercises	Muscle group	Purpose
Arm and shoulder	_____	_____	_____
	_____	_____	_____
	_____	_____	_____
Trunk	_____	_____	_____
	_____	_____	_____
Legs	_____	_____	_____
	_____	_____	_____
Other:	_____		_____

Figure 16.4 Muscular fitness program planner.

Muscular Fitness Program Planner

Sport ___Basketball___

Position ___Forward___

Season ___Off-season___

Goals ___Strength and power___

Individual strengths ___Shooting___

Weak points ___Rebounding___

Body Part	Exercises	Muscle group	Purpose
Arm and shoulder	Lat pull-downs (with basketball)	Hands, arms, chest, and lats	Pull-down rebounds
	Bicep curl	Arm flexors	Rebounding
Trunk	Abdominal curl (machine)	Abdominals	Pull-down rebounds
	Back-ups	Lower back	Back strength
Legs	Leaper or power squats	Leg extension and jumping muscles	Sustained power for jumping
	Plyometrics (down jumping)	Leg extension and jumping muscles	Preload and jumping
	Hill (or stair) running	Leg extension and jumping muscles	Sustained power
	Rebounding and fast break drills		Sustained power and endurance in game situations

Note. When sufficient strength is acquired, shift to an endurance, power, or power-endurance program in the preseason (achieve power-endurance with 15-25 reps as fast as possible).

Figure 16.5 Sample muscular fitness program.

17

The Environment and Performance

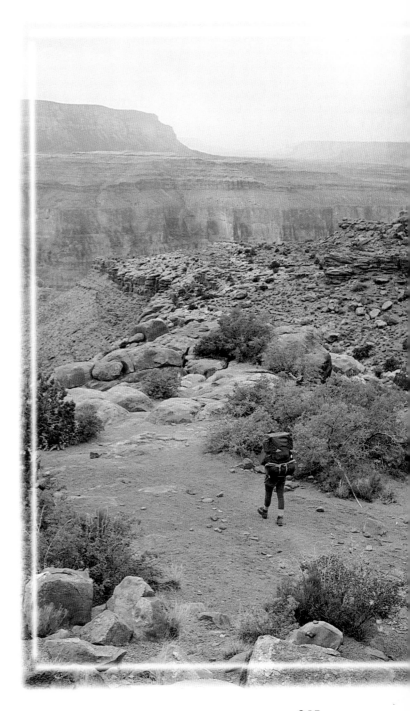

"No athlete is crowned but in the sweat of his brow."

St. Jerome

When I moved to Montana I fully expected to face a cold and sometimes hostile environment, and I looked forward to spending time at higher elevations. What I didn't expect was the potential for high temperatures in the summer months, and I certainly didn't expect to find air pollution, not in a state with only 800,000 residents spread out over 150,000 square miles (388,500 square kilometers) of open space. Over the years I've learned some tricks for coping with and even enjoying environmental extremes.

Environmental factors such as heat and cold, humidity, altitude, and even air pollution can have profound effects on health and performance. Failure to consider these effects can lead to serious problems, even death. On the other hand, it is entirely possible to adjust or acclimate to the environment, enabling you to perform well and comfortably under a wide range of conditions. Let's consider the problems caused by extremes of temperature, humidity, altitude, and air pollution to see how fitness and proper planning can minimize their effects.

■ This chapter will help you

- anticipate the effects of the environment on performance,
- take appropriate steps to minimize environmental effects, and
- understand how fitness enhances your ability to acclimatize and perform in difficult environments.

Temperature Regulation

The body's temperature-regulating mechanism consists of four parts:

- A regulating center located in the hypothalamus, an area at the base of the brain that serves as a thermostat to maintain body temperature at or near 37 degrees Celsius (98.6 degrees Fahrenheit)
- Heat and cold receptors located in the skin to sense changes in environmental temperature conditions
- Regulators such as muscles that increase body heat by shivering
- Vasomotor (nervous system) controls that constrict or dilate arterioles to conserve or lose body heat

The temperature-regulating center responds to the temperature of the blood flowing by the hypothalamus. If the blood cools, the thermostat sends information to conserve heat by constriction of blood vessels in the skin and the extremities. Some heat also can be generated by shivering.

If the blood temperature rises above the desired level (sometimes called a set point), the regulating center can cause dilation of cutaneous (skin) blood vessels and also stimulate the production of sweat. Consequently, blood is brought from the warmer core of the body to the surface, allowing heat loss by conduction, convection, and radiation as well as by evaporation of sweat from the surface of the skin. Complete evaporation of one liter of sweat leads to a heat loss of 580 calories. However, if the sweat drips off the body, little heat is lost.

Heat and cold receptors in the skin also aid in the maintenance of body temperature. The cold of the ski slopes will cause constriction of blood vessels, especially in the hands and feet. The extremities will stay cold until you elevate the body temperature, warm the blood, and reopen the blood vessels. This can best be done by vigorous exercise. Of course, you can put on more clothing or seek relief in the lodge.

The stifling heat of the tennis court will cause dilation of blood vessels that diverts a significant amount of blood from the muscles to the surface of the skin. The heart rate increases in an effort to maintain blood flow to the working muscles and the skin. Sweating will eventually reduce blood volume, and unless the water is replaced, your performance will suffer. If you persist in the activity and fail to replace the water loss, you may end up with heat exhaustion or heatstroke. So you are wise to listen to your body's call for rest, shade, and fluid replacement.

Individual differences in body fat, number of sweat glands, fitness level, and possibly gender may influence your response to heat.

- **Body fat:** Body fat serves as a layer of insulation beneath the surface of the skin. People with more subcutaneous fat may be better insulated from the cold, but are they less able to lose excess heat to the environment? Probably not, because the body learns to route blood around the fat for cooling purposes. Excess fat is a handicap in that it takes extra energy just to carry it around.

- **Sweat glands:** Each of us inherits a certain number and pattern of sweat glands. Because evaporative heat loss is the most important protection against heat stress, a good supply of active sweat glands is important. Like almost everything else, sweat glands respond to use. If you use them a lot, they become more efficient.

Fitness seems to enhance the ability to regulate body temperature during work in the heat.

- **Physical fitness:** Fitness seems to enhance the ability to regulate body temperature during work in the heat. It does so by lowering the temperature (set point) at which sweating begins. Thus fit individuals can work or play with lower heart rates and core temperatures than those of their unfit counterparts. Acclimatization further lowers the point at which sweating begins; therefore, the physically fit and heat-acclimated individual is even better prepared for work in the heat (Nadel 1977). And recent evidence indicates that fitness hastens the process of acclimatization.

- **Gender:** Men produce more sweat than women for a given increase in body temperature, perhaps too much. Women are efficient sweaters; production is more suited to the heat load, so they don't waste water. When men and women are compared on the same task, men seem better able to work in the heat; however, the difference is due to fitness, not gender. When the fitness level is the same or when the workload is equated (e.g., a given percentage of maximal oxygen intake), women are quite able to work in the heat. In several recent marathons, the women seemed to tolerate the heat as well as or better than many men, probably because they are more efficient sweaters.

Other factors that can influence your response to the heat are illness, medications, drugs, and alcohol. If you have been ill, your thermoregulatory system will take several days to recover. Many prescription and over-the-counter medications, as well as all recreational drugs and alcohol, can influence the body's response in a hot environment. If you are in doubt about medications or drugs, check with a physician or pharmacist before you risk exposure in a hot environment.

Exercising in the Heat

When exercise begins, the temperature-regulating center increases the body's usual set point, and the body temperature is allowed to increase. The rise in

Table 17.1   Conversion of Fahrenheit (F) to Celsius (C)

°F	°C
–40	–40
0	–18
32	0
50	10
72	22
85	29
98.6*	37
212	100

*Normal body temperature.

temperature depends on the intensity of exercise. In a moderate environment, the temperature will increase about 1 degree Celsius at 50 percent of the maximal oxygen intake, and will rise to about 39 degrees (a rise of two degrees Celsius) at the maximal level (above 102 degrees Fahrenheit; see table 17.1). This resetting of the core temperature during exercise can be viewed as an adjustment favorable to the enzyme activity within the muscles. It also serves to reduce the problem of heat dissipation. Under moderate environmental conditions, the methods of heat dissipation are not employed until the elevated set point has been reached.

In hot environments, we are able to maintain temporary thermal balance during exercise by virtue of circulatory adjustments and the evaporation of sweat. In a hot, dry environment, the body actually gains heat when the air temperature exceeds the temperature of the skin. Under these conditions, the evaporation of sweat allows the maintenance of thermal equilibrium. However, when the humidity also is high and evaporation cannot take place, heat is stored, the body temperature rises, and performance is severely impaired. Blood is diverted from muscles to the skin, blood volume is reduced via sweating, and water and electrolytes are lost in the sweat. Stroke volume declines, heart rate increases, and lactic acid accumulates. Blood may even begin to pool in the large veins, further reducing venous return and cardiac output. This hyperthermia, an alarming rise in body temperature, sets the stage for heat stress disorders, heat exhaustion, or even heatstroke, the potentially fatal collapse of the temperature-regulating mechanism (see "Heat Stress," p. 350).

Sweating

Because work capacity becomes impaired as water loss progresses, it is essential that the fluid be replaced.

In a normal day, we lose and must replace about 2.5 liters of water (one liter equals 1.057 quarts; one quart equals 0.946 liters). Of this water loss, about 0.7 liter comes from the lungs and skin (insensible water loss), 1.5 liters from the urine, 0.2 liters from the feces, and about 0.1 liter through perspiration. During heavy exercise in the heat, the water lost through sweating can exceed 2 liters per hour. Sweat production may amount to as much as 12 liters per day. Because work capacity becomes impaired as water loss progresses, it is essential that the fluid be replaced. Dehydration in excess of 3 to 5 percent of body weight leads to a marked decline in strength, endurance, and work capacity. Estimate 1 liter for each two-pound (.9-kilogram)

Highly fit individuals become acclimatized in four to five days, whereas sedentary subjects take twice as long. The best way to acclimatize is to work in the actual conditions (temperature and humidity) you'll have to endure. However, if you live in a cool climate and don't have a heat chamber in which to achieve acclimatization, high-intensity training can get you halfway there, probably because of the heat generated during vigorous effort. It helps to use a nonrubberized sweat suit to increase the temperature close to the skin. Fit individuals start to sweat at a lower body temperature, and they increase sweat production at a faster rate. Acclimatization helps move the set point for sweating even lower.

Less-fit individuals should acclimatize using periods of light to moderate activity in a hot environment, alternated with rest periods where fluid is replaced. Electrolytes can be replaced with commercial drinks or the saltshaker at meals, plus potassium-rich citrus fruits or bananas. The vitamin C in the citrus drinks may hasten the acclimatization process.

In summary, the prescription for exercise in a hot, humid environment includes the following advice:

- Wear porous, light-colored, loose-fitting clothing.
- Acclimatize to the expected environment and workload (i.e., do 50 percent the first day, 60 percent the second, and add 10 percent each day until you do 100 percent on the sixth day).
- Take 250 to 500 milligrams a day of vitamin C while acclimatizing.
- Always replace water and electrolytes.
- Find a cool place for rest periods.
- Always work or train with a partner.
- Don't be too proud to quit when you feel the symptoms of heat stress (dizziness, confusion, cramps, nausea, clammy skin).
- Keep a record of body weight during prolonged periods of work or training in the heat. Weigh in before and after exercise to gauge fluid loss. To check for day-to-day rehydration, weigh yourself in the morning, after toilet but before breakfast.
- Maintain aerobic fitness; the enhanced circulatory system and blood volume will help you work better in the heat, acclimate faster, and hold your acclimatization longer.

Follow these suggestions and you can join the "mad dogs and Englishmen" out in the midday sun.

Exercising in the Cold

Because of the metabolic heat generated during exercise, cold temperatures do not pose a threat similar to that posed by hot, humid conditions. But severe exposure to low temperatures and high winds can lead to frostbite, freezing, hypothermia, and even death. Constriction of blood vessels (vasoconstriction) increases the insulating capacity of the skin, but it also results in a marked reduction in the temperature of the extremities. It's almost as if the body is willing to lose a few fingers or toes to save the more important parts. Protective vasoconstriction often leads to severe discomfort in the fingers and toes. To relieve the pain, it is necessary to warm the affected area or raise the core temperature to allow reflexive return of blood to the extremities. Though shivering may cause some increase in temperature, gross muscular activity is far more effective in restoring heat to the troubled area. Because large muscle activity takes considerable energy, the cold-weather enthusiast must maintain a reserve of energy for use in emergencies. Excessive fatigue is the first step toward hypothermia and possible death.

Wind Chill

The wind chill describes the effect of wind speed on heat loss (see figure 17.3). A 10-degree Fahrenheit (minus 12-degree Celsius) reading is equivalent to minus 25 degrees Fahrenheit (minus 32 Celsius) when the wind speed is 20 miles (32.2 kilometers) per hour. Runners, skiers, and skaters can create their own wind chill. Skiing at 20 miles per hour on a 10-degree Fahrenheit day is equivalent to minus 25 degrees. And if the skier is moving into a wind, the effect is even worse. When possible, run, ski, or skate away from the wind. If you must face into the wind on a cold day, be sure to cover exposed flesh, including earlobes and nose, and be on the lookout for frostbite.

Wind speed (mph)	Actual thermometer reading (°F)												
	50	40	30	20	10	0	−10	−20	−30	−40	−50	−60
	Equivalent temperature (°F)												
Calm	50	40	30	20	10	0	−10	−20	−30	−40	−50	−60
5	48	37	27	16	6	−5	−15	−26	−36	−47	−57	−68
10	40	28	16	4	−9	−21	−33	−46	−58	−70	−83	−95
15	36	22	9	−5	−18	−36	−45	−58	−72	−85	−99	−112
20	32	18	4	−10	−25	−39	−53	−67	−82	−96	−110	−124
25	30	16	0	−15	−29	−44	−59	−74	−88	−104	−118	−133
30	28	13	−2	−18	−33	−48	−63	−79	−94	−109	−125	−140
35	27	11	−4	−20	−35	−49	−67	−82	−98	−113	−129	−145
40	26	10	−6	−21	−37	−53	−69	−85	−100	−116	−132	−148

Little Danger (for properly clothed person)   Increasing Danger   Great Danger

Danger from freezing of exposed flesh

Figure 17.3 Wind-chill index.

Reprinted from Sharkey 1974.

Frostbite

Frostbite is damage to the skin resulting from exposure to extreme cold or wind chill. As you can see on the wind-chill index, there is little danger of frostbite at temperatures above 20 degrees Fahrenheit (minus 7 degrees Celsius). A temperature or wind chill of minus 20 degrees Fahrenheit (minus 29 degrees Celsius) seems necessary to produce the condition.

At first, frostbite appears as a patch of pale or white skin, due to the constriction of blood vessels in the area. After mild frostbite, the skin appears red and swollen when the blood returns. In severe frostbite, the skin may appear purple or black after it is warmed. Immersion in warm (not hot) water will hasten the return of blood to the area. Do not massage the affected part. Protect the groin and other sensitive areas to avoid the excruciating pain that occurs when circulation returns. And if your feet become frostbitten on a winter outing, do not remove your boots to warm your feet. Your feet could swell and you wouldn't be able to put your boots back on. Walk or ski out before removing your boots and warming your feet.

If you're worried about freezing the delicate tissues of the lungs during cold-weather exercise, don't. Cold air may make your breathing uncomfortable because it is so dry, but there is little danger of damage to the tissue. The respiratory system has a remarkable ability to warm and humidify air. Humans tolerate air temperatures well below minus 20 degrees Fahrenheit (minus 29 Celsius) without damage. The cold air is warmed to above 32 degrees Fahrenheit (0 degrees Celsius) before it reaches the bronchi. However, when the temperature goes below minus 20, you are advised to modify or curtail your exercise plans. The danger to earlobes, nose, fingers, and toes is great, and at much lower temperatures respiratory tract damage is possible, though unlikely. Very cold air constricts airways and makes vigorous effort difficult.

If you're worried about freezing the delicate tissues of the lungs during cold-weather exercise, don't.

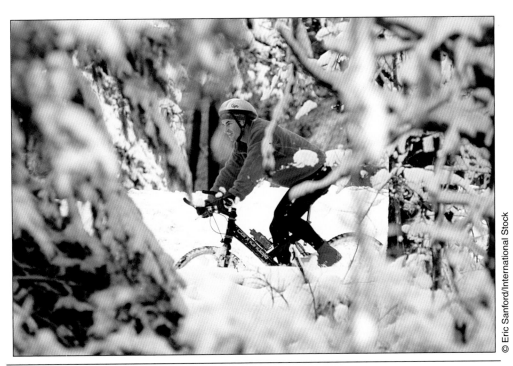

Don't allow cold temperatures to limit your activity.

© Eric Sanford/International Stock

Hypothermia

When your body begins to lose heat faster than it can be produced, you are undergoing exposure. Prolonged exertion leads to progressive muscular fatigue. Shivering and vasoconstriction are attempts to preserve body heat and the temperature of vital organs. Exhaustion of energy stores and neuromuscular impairment lead to the virtual termination of activity. As exposure continues and additional body heat is lost, the cold reaches the brain; you lose judgment and the ability to reason. Your speech becomes slow and slurred, you lose control of your hands, walking becomes clumsy, and you want to lie down and rest. Don't do it! You are hypothermic. Your core temperature is dropping, and without treatment you will lose consciousness and die.

You may be surprised to learn that most hypothermia cases occur in air temperatures above 30 degrees Fahrenheit (minus 1 degree Celsius). Cold water, wind chill, and fatigue combine to set the stage for hypothermia. Avoid the problem by staying dry. If you become wet, dry off as soon as possible. Be aware of the wind chill and how wind refrigerates wet clothing. During a cold-weather hike or ski tour, take off layers of clothing before you perspire, and put them back on as you begin to cool. Eat and rest often to maintain your energy level. Stop or make camp when you still have energy; don't wait until the situation is critical.

If someone exhibits the symptoms of hypothermia, transport the victim to a medical facility as quickly as possible. The heart may begin to fibrillate during rewarming, and emergency equipment will be needed. If immediate transport isn't possible, or if the case isn't severe, do the following:

- Get the victim out of the wind and rain.
- Remove all wet clothing.
- Provide dry clothing; warm drinks; and a warm, dry sleeping bag for a mildly impaired victim.
- If the victim is only semiconscious, try to keep the person awake, and put him or her, unclothed, in a sleeping bag with another person.
- Build a fire.

Cold-Weather Clothing

For extended periods of outdoor exertion when you'll be away from protective shelter and central heating, dress in layers. Layers of clothing provide an insulating barrier of air and can be peeled off as your temperature rises and put back on as it falls. Wool is one of the best fabrics to wear for under and outer garments. It doesn't have the insulating value of dry down, but it is far better than down when wet.

Physiologists rate the insulating value of clothing in "Clo" units, with one Clo unit being equivalent to the clothing that will maintain comfort at a room temperature of 70 degrees Fahrenheit, or 21 degrees Celsius (roughly equivalent to a cotton shirt and slacks). Table 17.2 and figure 17.4 illustrate how the insulating

Table 17.2 Comfort Data

Effective temperature (°F)	Thickness of insulation required for comfort (in.)		
	Sleeping	Light work	Heavy work
40 (4°C)	1.5 (3.8 cm)	0.8 (2.0 cm)	.20 (0.5 cm)
20 (−7°C)	2.0 (5 cm)	1.0 (2.5 cm)	.27 (0.70 cm)
0 (−18°C)	2.5 (6.4 cm)	1.3 (3.3 cm)	.35 (0.90 cm)
−20 (−29°C)	3.0 (7.6 cm)	1.6 (4.1 cm)	.40 (1.0 cm)
−40 (−40°C)	3.5 (8.9 cm)	1.9 (4.8 cm)	.48 (1.2 cm)

These figures are approximate but are a good base for an average healthy person.

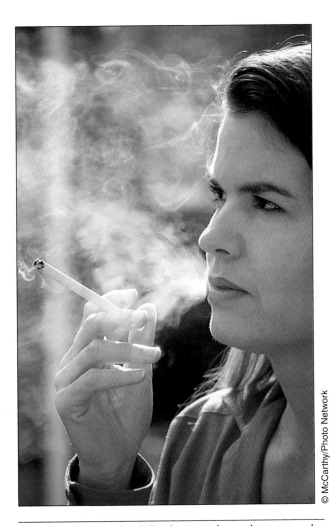

© McCarthy/Photo Network

Secondhand smoke kills thousands and impairs the health of hundreds of thousands of children every year.

as high as 166 parts per million inside an automobile with windows closed. It wouldn't be long before the nonsmoker felt symptoms of distress, headache, and nausea. The smoker, however, has become less sensitive and wouldn't be bothered. We should continue efforts to restrict smoking in public places. Assert your right to a smoke-free atmosphere.

In addition to bronchitis, emphysema, and cancer, the nicotine, carbon monoxide, and other toxic compounds in cigarette smoke combine to dramatically increase the risk of heart disease. Women should never smoke while pregnant, and because environmental tobacco smoke (or secondhand smoke) causes asthma and other breathing problems for children, parents should never smoke in the house or in the car. Smoking contributes to accidents, illness, and disabling injuries, and smoking costs business and industry billions in additional health care, worker's compensation, and cleaning costs.

Respirable Particulate

The soot that clogs the air above major cities contains a range of particles. Large particles are trapped in the upper respiratory tract. The human respiratory system has a remarkable ability to cleanse itself via the action of the ciliary escalator, which sweeps smaller particles upward so they can be expectorated. When the particulate load is great or sustained, as in smoking or urban pollution, the ciliary mechanism can break down.

Some particles are small enough to find their way deep into the lung. These respirable particles are rendered more dangerous because of carcinogenic compounds that sometimes attach to the particles. A study of six American cities showed that mortality (death) rates were strongly associated with fine particulate pollution (<2.5 micrometers). These products of combustion—coming from industry, diesel and other engines, and residential wood burning—penetrate indoors to foul the air we breathe. Though air pollution was positively associated with death from lung cancer and cardiopulmonary disease, mortality rates were most strongly associated with cigarette smoking (Dockery et al. 1993).

Many other pollutants are known to irritate respiratory passages; cause bronchitis, allergies, and asthma; contribute to heart and chronic obstructive lung disease; and cause lung and other cancers. Ozone, formaldehyde, benzene, asbestos, sulfur dioxide, nitrous oxides, and other by-products from internal combustion engines are a few of the hundreds of compounds considered toxic to humans (for information visit **www.epa.gov**, the Web site of the U.S. Environmental Protection Agency, or **www.niosh.gov**, the Web site for the National Institute for Occupational Safety and Health).

We must continue the fight for clean air so our activities need not be regulated in accordance with the air pollution index, and our enjoyment of physical activity need not be compromised by humankind's mistreatment of the environment. In the meantime, avoid exercise in obviously dangerous areas (along expressways, near industrial pollution) and when air pollution warnings are in effect. That doesn't mean you shouldn't exercise; just find a way to avoid the pollution. And be sure to add your voice to the growing fight against all forms of pollution, including the worst of all, the cigarette.

Summary

In this chapter I've outlined the problems encountered in different environments and provided practical advice on how to minimize the problems and maximize performance and enjoyment. Solutions range from improving fitness and acclimatization to dressing properly and maintaining hydration and energy. Fitness, while especially important in the heat, improves performance in all environments. Acclimatization is necessary for heat and altitude and useful in the cold. Fluid replacement is critical in the heat, but it is also extremely important in the cold and at altitude, where considerable fluid is lost during breathing. The maintenance of energy levels is essential to prolonged performance in any environment. Finally, proper clothing is required to cope with the demands of the environment.

But what of air pollution? What can be done to minimize its effects? The answers are simple: Minimize exposure and maintain your immune system with regular exercise, rest, and good nutrition. Include immune-friendly foods in your diet (see chapter 11) and use antioxidant supplements to counter the free radicals found in pollutants. Minimize exposure by exercising where or when pollution levels are lowest. If you are particularly sensitive to pollutants or allergens, you may want to use a dust mask to filter particles, or a mask impregnated with activated charcoal to absorb pollutants. Unfortunately, simple masks do not remove carbon monoxide, so avoid high-traffic areas during exercise.

PART VI

Vitality and Longevity

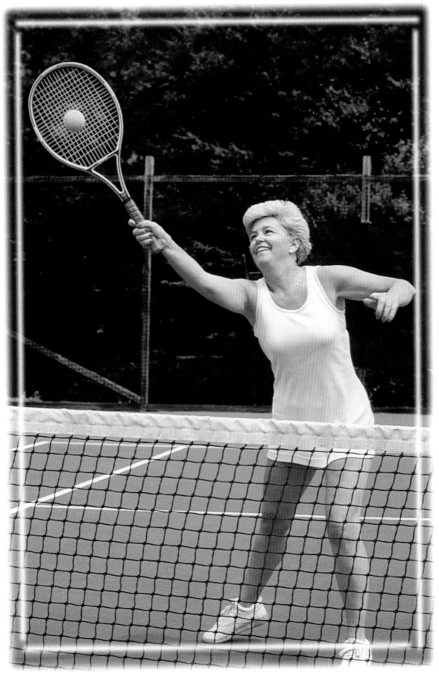

The prevailing view of aging is a dreary one, depicting a life of limits and ailments, a vicious cycle with loss of function, frailty, and failure. Fortunately, you do not have to accept this tragic opera as your script. If you are willing to adopt the appropriate lifestyle, you will be able to take command of your role, to write and perform an epic that features a long and satisfying life.

The final chapters of this book are designed to help you develop the daily habits, psychosocial skills, and other behaviors that contribute to a happy, healthy, and vigorous life. Daily habits are an indispensable part of your life, and the appropriate habits contribute to health and the quality of life. Psychosocial skills are necessary for a full and complete life. Chapter 19 provides ways to utilize psychology to help motivate and maintain your commitment to regular moderate physical activity.

The goal is to be vigorous and fully involved throughout life, to live each stage to the fullest. In return for your efforts you will retain the vitality and mobility needed for a full, independent life, and you may even live longer. But the most compelling outcome of the active life is that you'll add life to your years, not just years to your life. Stated simply, you'll extend the prime of life.

18

Age, Activity, and Vitality

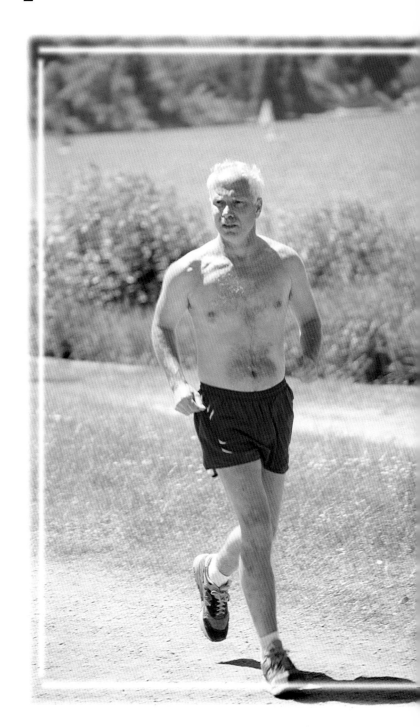

"The daily habits of people have a great deal more to do with what makes them sick and when they die than all the influences of medicine."

Lester Breslow, MD

Age tells little about your health, your appearance, your fitness, or your ability to perform. Though aging inevitably leads to death, it does so at different rates for different people, depending on heredity and on personal decisions on how you choose to age.

Sometime after the peak reproductive years, when the direct evolutionary advantage has passed, virtually all tissues and organs begin to age. Parents remain important, at least until the child becomes a young adult, and grandparents serve to pass on wisdom or to assist the parents. But when a person reaches the 70s there is little biological justification to continue life, and indeed, life expectancies range from 78 to 79 for women and 73 to 74 for men. But life expectancies, which have risen throughout the past century, tell only part of the story.

▌ This chapter will help you

- differentiate life expectancy from life span,
- understand how activity and other habits influence longevity,
- see how fitness influences your physiological age, and
- understand how activity and fitness extend the prime of life.

Life Span

Life expectancy has gone up in proportion to declines in infant mortality and infectious diseases. But the attainable life span, the age attainable in a life free of serious accident or illness, has not changed noticeably in the past 200 years. In other words, we are not living longer; we are avoiding premature death. Survival curves point to a theoretically attainable life span of about 85 years, with a standard deviation of 4 years (figure 18.1). Thus 68 percent of the population have the potential to live between 81 and 89 years (85 plus or minus 4 years), and 95 percent of deaths from natural causes would fall between 77 and 93 years (85 plus or minus two standard deviations, or 8 years). Rare indeed are the individuals who live beyond 97 years, more than three standard deviations above the mean. The oldest documented life spans are in the neighborhood of 120 years (Fries and Crapo 1981).

Postponement of chronic illness has extended the period of adult vigor, so life remains physically, emotionally, and intellectually vigorous until shortly before its close (figure 18.2). Many of the factors believed to be associated with age can be modified with appropriate behaviors, including heart and lung function, bone density, blood pressure, and cholesterol. People who choose not to age rapidly can reduce morbidity and extend the vigorous years by living an active, healthy life (Fries and Crapo 1981). On the other hand, those who decide to age rapidly are destined to become a burden on family, health care, and community support systems.

Earlier I quoted studies that indicate an increase in longevity for those who lead the active life. Activity adds life to your years as well as years to your life! Unfortunately, as some have said, the years you add all come at the end. And it has been suggested that the years you add are about equal to the time spent in exercise. Can that be true? One study found at least a two-year increase in life

Activity adds life to your years as well as years to your life! Unfortunately, as some have said, the years you add all come at the end.

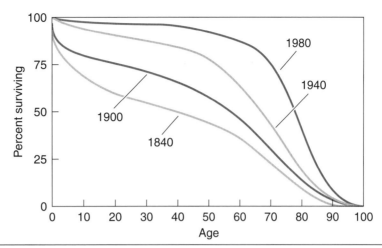

Figure 18.1 Survival curves. With less infant mortality and trauma (accidental death), more people survive to the attainable life expectancy, 85 years. With good health habits, more are able to postpone chronic debilitating illness, to remain vigorous until the last years or months of life.

Adapted from *Vital Statistics of the United States*, 1977 (vol. 2, sec. 5). DHEW Publication PHS 80-1104, National Center for Health Statistics.

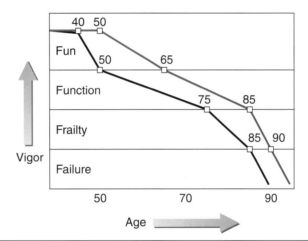

Figure 18.2 Vigor and the active life. Active living extends the periods of fun and function and shortens the time of frailty and failure.

expectancy associated with activity. If you exercise one hour every day for 40 years you'll spend 14,560 hours engaged in exercise. Divide that number by 24 hours per day, and you get 607 days, or 1.67 years, somewhat less than the two years or more you'll earn. Of course, you will enjoy the time you spend in exercise, recreation, and sport, and you will extend the years of fun and function, the prime of life.

Aging

Theories of aging are many, including those dealing with gene defects or chromosomal damage, errors in protein synthesis, and limits to the number of cell divisions (the Hayflick limit). Other factors associated with aging include caloric intake and specific nutrients.

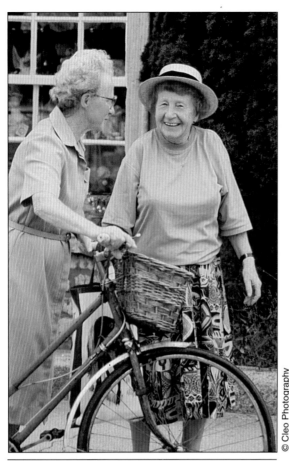

© Cleo Photography

Exercise will extend the prime of life.

What is surprising is the realization that the rate of decline or senescence is not fixed but variable, subject to considerable modification.

• **Caloric restriction:** Animal studies have shown that eating fewer calories (up to 40 percent less) can extend survival time dramatically (28 percent in one study) when adult animals were put on a low-protein diet (Miller and Payne 1968). Some researchers have felt that the most important factors determining life span were those that influenced body fatness. Animals fed fewer calories also had a lower tumor incidence and less chronic disease (Comfort 1979). When Alexander Leaf studied healthy old people in three remote parts of the world he found their diets low in calories and fat (1973). Leaf believed that the low-calorie diet, combined with regular activity and a productive and respected role in society, contributed to good health and long life.

• **Free radicals:** One theory of aging holds that so-called free radicals (reactive molecules with one or more unpaired electrons) prove toxic to vulnerable tissues. In the biologic world, life span is inversely related to metabolic rate. Exercise produces free radicals that could harm the body. But moderate activity enhances antioxidant protection and the immune system. Chronic heavy exertion may produce an excess of free radicals, raise the risk of heart disease, and depress the immune response (Demopolus et al. 1986). The role of free radicals in exercise and aging requires more study. In the meantime, vitamins C and E and beta-carotene are believed to provide some protection against these potentially toxic by-products of oxidative metabolism.

At present no single theory explains the decline that occurs with age. What is surprising is the realization that the rate of decline or senescence is not fixed but variable, subject to considerable modification. What has emerged is a list of modifiable aspects of aging, markers that are subject to changes brought about by one's personal decisions and behaviors (table 18.1).

A definite pattern emerges from a consideration of the modifiable aspects of aging, a pattern that points to the importance of daily habits as the way to improve your health span, your active life expectancy.

Health Habits

Since 1962, researchers at the Human Population Laboratory of the California Department of Health have studied the relationship of health to various behaviors or habits. Health and longevity are associated with the following:

• Adequate sleep (seven to eight hours per day)
• A good breakfast
• Regular meals—avoid snacks
• Weight control

Table 18.1 Modifiable and Non-Modifiable Aspects of Aging

Aging marker	Personal decision/behavior
Modifiable aspects	
Cardiac output	Exercise
Glucose tolerance	Exercise, diet, weight control
Osteoporosis	Weight-bearing exercise, diet
Pulmonary function	Exercise, nonsmoking
Blood pressure	Exercise, diet, weight control
Endurance and strength	Exercise
Reaction time	Training, practice
Cholesterol	Diet, weight control, exercise
Arterial wall rigidity	Diet, exercise
Intelligence and memory	Training, practice
Skin aging	Avoid sun
Non-modifiable aspects	
Elasticity of skin	Avoid sun, nonsmoking
Graying, thinning of hair	
Kidney reserve	
Cataracts	

Adapted from Fries and Crapo 1981.

- Not smoking cigarettes
- Moderate alcohol consumption
- Regular exercise

The study found that men could add 11 years to their lives and women 7 years, just by following six of the habits (Breslow and Enstrom 1980). Let's examine each practice to see if it fits your current lifestyle. Then you can decide if changes are in order.

Sleep

When men or women sleep six hours or less per night, they are not as healthy as when they sleep seven or eight hours. Those who sleep nine hours or more are slightly below average in health. Thus seven to eight hours of sleep is most favorable, and, as you might expect, too little sleep is more of a problem than too much.

Sleep is characterized by alternating stages. One stage involves rapid eye movements (REM) and changes in heart rate, blood pressure, and muscle tone.

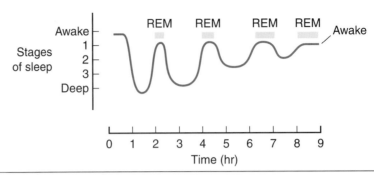

Figure 18.3 The stages of sleep.

This stage may serve as a rest period for the inhibitory nerve cells of the brain. It usually is accompanied by dreams, and if it is interrupted we become anxious and irritable. This REM sleep constitutes about 20 percent of the night's total, whereas deeper or quieter periods provide the rest necessary for recovery from fatigue. If you miss some sleep one night, the body will not make any serious attempt to recover the sleep deprivation. However, if a substantial amount of the loss is REM sleep, more REM sleep will occur on subsequent nights (figure 18.3). Going without sleep seems to impair creative capabilities, which suggests that another function of sleep is to restore a cerebral cortex fatigued by consciousness.

Moderate physical activity seems to enhance the ability to fall into deep sleep without altering the time spent in REM sleep. Too little or too much exercise appears to result in sleep disturbance, and significant sleep loss seems to suppress the immune system.

Breakfast

In the California study, those who ate breakfast almost every day experienced better health than those who ate breakfast some of the time (Breslow and Enstrom 1980). Furthermore, a good breakfast may be a prerequisite to good performance in work and sport. Breakfast often comes 12 hours after the evening meal, so you can see why it is important for energy and cellular metabolism. A few researchers suggest that breakfast should be the largest and most important meal of the day, and everyone agrees that it should include more than a cup of coffee and a doughnut.

Regular Meals

Erratic eaters have poorer health than those who eat regular meals. Those who seldom or never eat between meals have better health than those who regularly eat between meals. Unfortunately, this study did not compare the health status of those who eat smaller but more numerous nutritious meals, but it does indicate the effects of erratic eating behavior and snacking. We can only guess at the content of the between-meal snacks, but chances are that they were toxic foods, high in simple sugars and saturated fat and low in nutrients (Breslow and Enstrom 1980).

Weight Control

When weight is more than 20 percent above or more than 10 percent below the desirable weight, health status declines. For example, if your desirable weight is listed as 150 pounds (68 kilograms), your health status is most favorable when you maintain your weight between 135 pounds (61.2 kilograms; minus 10 percent) and 180 pounds (81.6 kilograms; plus 20 percent), a broad margin of error indeed. It would be interesting to compare the effects on health of low body weight (more than 10 percent below desirable) due to malnutrition, illness, or smoking, and low weight due to habitual vigorous exercise. Personal observations indicate that a low body weight associated with vigorous exercise and good nutrition is at least as healthy as being at or above the desirable weight.

Smoking

Smoking, especially cigarette smoking, is dangerous to your health. If you don't smoke, don't start. If you do, stop. It could be the best thing you ever did for yourself. And if you can't stop for your own health, think of loved ones, especially children, who are exposed to your habit. Secondhand tobacco smoke is responsible for asthma and respiratory problems for many thousands of children, not to mention lung cancers. Is quitting worth the trouble? Data from numerous studies show that quitting has many benefits, including better oxygen-carrying capacity, lower blood pressure, improved night vision, and increased effectiveness of prescription drugs. And though some diseases, such as emphysema, cannot be reversed, others seem to repair with time. Repair time for smoking-induced illnesses include 10 years for heart disease and 10 to 15 years for cancer. Quit today and help make the nation smoke-free.

Alcohol

Poor health is associated with heavy alcohol consumption (five or more drinks at one sitting). Those who never drink and those who drink moderately (one to two drinks a day for men, one to three per *week* for women) enjoy the same level of good health. The French Paradox ponders why the French seem to tolerate rich foods without an increase in heart disease. The answer may lie in the regular consumption of wine. Some studies show that those who drink one or two alcoholic drinks daily have a lower risk of heart disease, perhaps because alcohol is associated with higher levels of HDL cholesterol (Gaziano et al. 1993). This should not be construed as a broad endorsement of alcoholic consumption. Some level of alcoholic consumption, if continued for a sufficient period, may lead to degenerative effects on the liver, even when nutrition is adequate. The best advice is to drink moderately (one to two drinks per day for men, one every other day for women), or don't drink at all. And no, you cannot save your daily drinks for a weekend binge.

Regular Activity

Researchers in the California study compared the health benefits of five types of activity: active sports, swimming or long walks, garden work, physical exercises, and hunting and fishing. Only hunting and fishing (seasonal and infrequent) were *not* associated with improved health. For all the others, those who participated most often experienced the best physical health. The best health was associated with active sports, followed by swimming or walking, physical exercise, and gardening. Lowest death rates were recorded for those who were often active in sports, and the highest rates were for those who chose not to engage in any exercise.

In summary, physical health, longevity, and the rate of aging are associated with your daily health habits and your lifestyle. These habits have more to do with your health and longevity than all the influences of medicine. The California study indicated that a man of 55 years who follows all seven health habits has the same health status as a person 25 to 30 years younger who follows fewer than two. Moreover, the researchers found a positive relationship between physical and mental health (Breslow and Enstrom 1980). You know that an association or relationship between variables does not imply cause and effect, that good physical health doesn't necessarily cause good mental health, but you are probably familiar with psychosomatic illnesses and should realize that the opposite effects are possible. A healthy body is an important aid to good mental health, and you can help maintain physical health by following the recommended health habits.

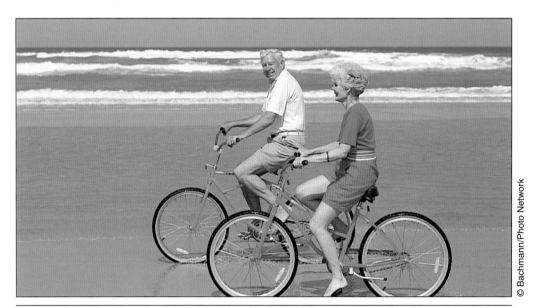

Those who age successfully engage in daily routines that require activity.

Longevity

One key to longevity, to what it takes to live well beyond normal life expectancy, is your lifestyle. Observations of healthy older individuals (aged 75 years and over) provide intriguing insights into the personality traits and living habits associated with long-term survival.

The following characteristics are associated with longevity:

- **Moderation:** Moderation is a common denominator in all phases of life, including diet, vices, work, and physical activity. Long-term survival in a footrace or the human race depends on pacing.

- **Flexibility:** Psychological flexibility implies the ability to bend but not break, to accept change, to avoid rigid habits.

- **Challenge:** Accept challenges; create them if necessary; don't allow life to become too easy. But when a challenge becomes too great, say so, and seek an alternative.

Initiating Behavior

Early success is associated with reasonable expectations and goals, gradual change, appropriate reinforcement, social support, and cognitive strategies (relaxation, dissociation). Relax during activity by focusing on your breathing.

Relaxation

Sit in a comfortable chair in a quiet room and repeat a simple sound (mantra) such as "easy" each time you exhale. Concentration on the breathing and the mantra masks disturbing thoughts, and the body begins to relax. As you become more proficient with the technique, you may achieve a transcendent state of relaxation, clear thought, imagery, well-being, and openness. In time you'll be able to use the skill during activity and sport. Meditation is not a substitute for exercise; it will not induce the many physiological changes that result from regular activity. On the other hand, some find activity to be as effective as meditation in the achievement of relaxation.

Dissociation involves diverting attention from how you feel during exercise by focusing on other topics or conversation with a partner. For some people, the first 20 minutes of activity are the hardest, until pain-killing endorphins kick in. Similarly, the first few weeks of a new program are the toughest. So it helps to have ways to cope until appreciable changes become evident or until you become addicted. Behavior therapy seems to work for difficult cases.

Behavior Therapy

This approach provides a way to identify a desired behavior and to make progress toward its acquisition. The essentials are threefold:

1. Identify the behavior you wish to modify (e.g., physical activity), and maintain an accurate record of your current behavior. Maintain a weeklong record of all your physical activity (figure 19.2). Include the intensity and duration of your involvement, and complete the cognitive question for fitness training and recreational activities.

2. Analyze the current behavior, and then plan needed modifications. Do you need to burn more calories, to increase intensity, or do specific training (e.g., muscular fitness)? Plan appropriate modifications to meet your needs and interests. For example, you could increase your activity to meet the CDC/ACSM guidelines: 30 minutes or more of moderate-intensity physical activity most days of the week.

3. Develop a contract with specific goals and a schedule of rewards to reinforce the new behavior (figure 19.3). Use activity benchmarks (minutes or miles [or kilometers] per day or week), weight loss, or other indicators of successful adoption of the new activity. A tangible, universally accepted reward such as money seems to work for most of us. Spend the reward immediately, or save it for something you really want but might otherwise not purchase. Don't worry about the expense; the new behavior will save more than the cost of the reward in medical and other expenses. In time the behavior will become a healthy habit, and you will be able to focus on new goals or new behaviors (e.g., weight control, time management).

Daily Activity Log

Date _____

Time	Place	Exercise	Intensity	Duration	What were your thoughts during exercise?

Note. Include all forms of physical activity, including work, walking, and household chores.

Score	Intensity	Score	Duration
5	Sustained heavy breathing and perspiration	4	Over 30 min
4	Intermittent heavy breathing and perspiration—as in tennis	3	20 to 30 min
3	Moderately heavy—as in recreational sports and cycling	2	10 to 20 min
2	Moderate—as in volleyball, softball	1	Under 10 min
1	Light—as in fishing, walking		

Figure 19.2 Daily activity log.

Activity Reinforcement Schedule

Date	Activity	Distance or time	Reward[a]	Total
____	_____			
____	_____			
____	_____			
____	_____			
____	_____	_____		_____
____	_____			
____	_____			
____	_____			
____	_____			
____	_____			
____	_____	_____		_____
____	_____			
____	_____			
____	_____			
____	_____			
____	_____	_____		_____
____	_____			
____	_____			
____	_____			
____	_____			
Total for month		_____		_____

Note. Daily reward—for meeting activity goal (e.g., 2 mi); weekly reward—for meeting activity goal (e.g., 12 mi); monthly reward—for meeting activity goal (e.g., 50 mi; improved fitness score). Adjust goals as fitness improves.

[a]Rewards: daily—a small monetary award (e.g., $1) or a cool drink; weekly—a larger monetary reward (e.g., $5) or a special favor (e.g., movie); monthly—a substantial monetary reward (e.g., $20) or a very special favor (e.g., concert, dinner out). Rewards can be saved for a special purpose (e.g., new warm-up outfit, tennis racquet).

Figure 19.3 Activity reinforcement schedule.

Maintenance

Adherence to a newly adopted behavior can be difficult; 50 percent of participants drop out of exercise programs within the first year. Certain strategies help to improve the odds of success (Taylor and Miller 1993). Activity is continued if

- it meets a need,
- it is fun,
- there is social support, and
- there is evidence of change.

To ensure lifelong participation, the individual must move from extrinsic to intrinsic motivation; must become self-sufficient, independent of the instructor and the setting; and must develop strategies to deal with factors that threaten continued participation. Work, illness, or family crises may interrupt but must never terminate participation in regular moderate activity.

Develop a network of support systems to help you guarantee adherence. Support is available from family and friends, interest groups, professionals, clubs, programs, publications, and organizations.

- **Family:** My wife and I provide support by taking a sincere interest in each other's activity, and we often participate together. Family gifts are often selected to encourage or enhance participation, and trips often revolve around a shared experience, such as hiking, canoeing, skiing, or golf.

- **Friends:** Most of my longtime friends are those who share my interests. The shared interests are the foundation of the relationship, and the glue that holds it together. Their presence gets me out and keeps me going. Together we do more than any of us would do alone.

- **Interest groups:** I have access to hiking, skiing, and running clubs, and more. The local canoe-racing group welcomes neophytes to join their Wednesday evening training sessions. If you can't find a group with your interests, start one.

- **Professionals:** From personal trainers to fitness and sport instructors, a wide array of help is available. Seek experts out for advice and for motivation. Get professional instruction to improve your performance and enjoyment of skiing or other recreational sports.

- **Clubs:** Join a health and fitness club, and you'll gain access to equipment; instruction; and an added bonus, the social support of fellow members. Club-based programs often succeed when home-based programs fail because of social and psychological support.

- **Programs:** Take advantage of your workplace wellness program and become involved in new activities. The wellness program at the university where I work has provided me with weightlifting, swimming, in-line skating, slide boards, ski clinics, and many other classes. Our campus recreation program has welcomed me on winter ski trips and in canoe and kayak classes.

- **Publications:** Many books are available to help you maintain or expand your interests. Magazines cater to general (*Outside*) or specific interests (*Backpacker*). Videos and computer programs on compact disc provide instruction in everything from golf to mountain biking.

- **Organizations:** The American College of Sports Medicine (ACSM) provides information and publications on fitness, exercise science, and sports medicine. ACSM also publishes position papers on a wide range of topics (**www.acsm.org**). Sport organizations such as the United States Tennis Association provide sport-specific pamphlets, instruction, and tournaments.

Sometimes a new piece of equipment will revive interest in an activity. For example, an adjustable ski pole has increased my interest in and enjoyment of backcountry hiking. The pole aids uphill travel, relieves aging knees on the downhills, and provides balance in crossing logs and streams. Sporting goods stores and equipment catalogs provide ways to make activity more pleasurable. Take advantage of these and other support systems to ensure a lifelong involvement in physical activity.

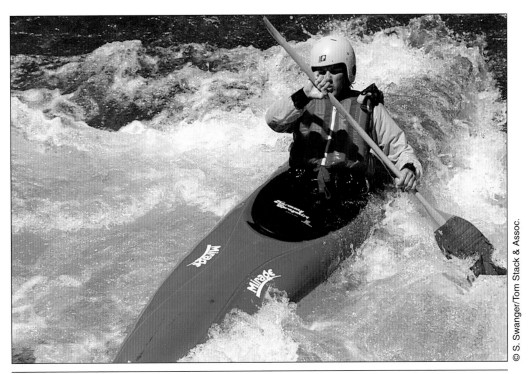

© S. Swanger/Tom Stack & Assoc.

A new sport or piece of equipment will add interest and enjoyment and bolster participation in the active life.

Relapse

It is not uncommon for participants to relapse, to slip back to inactivity after an initial change for the better. Relapse occurs for many reasons, ranging from emotional and social to physical. Because the event is so common, you should not let it bother you. It is part of the process of change, for athletes as well as newcomers. In dieting, relapse is par for the course. The question is, what can you do to prevent or recover from relapse? One approach calls for a planned relapse, just to test the reaction when instructor support is available. To date, most relapse-prevention programs have been labor-intensive, teaching how to anticipate and cope with relapse using strategies we have already discussed, such as behavior therapy and goal setting. Most have yielded modest results.

My suggestion is to search for intrinsic motivation and to strive for internal control. Free yourself from the need for external validation from fitness instructors. Their responsibility is to lead you to a level of independence where you will no longer rely on them for information or encouragement. Wean yourself from dependence on their motivation and control. Then develop your own approach to relapse prevention. Build the social support and emotional climate you need to keep going. Don't depend on one activity; be ready to adapt in the event of injury or chronic illness. When relapse comes, and it will, return to your goals, to behavior therapy, and to your support systems. People who develop behavioral or cognitive strategies, such as positive self-talk, are more successful at coping with relapse (Willis and Campbell 1992). Devise your own solution, and you'll be better prepared for the future. But if all else fails, don't hesitate to consult a professional.

The Active Personality

Do activity and improved fitness influence the personality, or are some personality types more likely to be active? Personality is a frame of reference used by psychologists in the study of behavior. More than a mask but less than reality; it is a product of heredity and the environment, usually studied with paper-and-pencil tests or in-depth interviews, but it has never really been defined or measured. That should not deter scientists in their search. The day may come when we will be able to define and measure this elusive concept of personality and thus understand, predict, or even improve behavior and health.

Cattell suggests that one's personality indicates what he or she will do when in a given mood and placed in a given situation. He developed the Cattell 16 Personality Factor Questionnaire, a personality test used widely by researchers (Cattell, Eber, and Tatsuoka 1970). The test, typical of the paper-and-pencil approach, presumes to score the subject on each of 16 factors, or personality "traits" (see table 19.1). Assuming this approach is valid, let's use it to consider how activity and personality are related.

Using the Cattell questionnaire, studies of the personalities of middle-aged men have shown that highly fit subjects are more unconventional, composed, secure, easygoing, emotionally stable, adventurous, and higher in intelligence than the low-fitness subjects. The most pronounced personality differences were those related to emotional stability and security. However, the presence of

Table 19.1 Cattell's 16 Personality Factors

Low score description	Personality factors	High score description
Aloof, cold	A	Warm, sociable
Dull, low capacity	B	Bright, intelligent
Emotional, unstable	C	Mature, calm
Submissive, mild	E	Dominant, aggressive
Glum, silent	F	Enthusiastic, talkative
Casual, undependable	G	Conscientious, persistent
Timid, shy	H	Adventurous, "thick-skinned"
Tough, realistic	I	Sensitive, effeminate
Trustful, adaptable	L	Suspecting, jealous
Conventional, practical	M	Bohemian, unconcerned
Simple, awkward	N	Sophisticated, polished
Confident, unshakable	Q	Insecure, anxious
Conservative, accepting	Q_1	Experimenting, critical
Dependent, imitative	Q_2	Self-sufficient, resourceful
Lax, unsure	Q_3	Controlled, exact
Phlegmatic, composed	Q_4	Tense, excitable

20

Activity and the Quality of Life

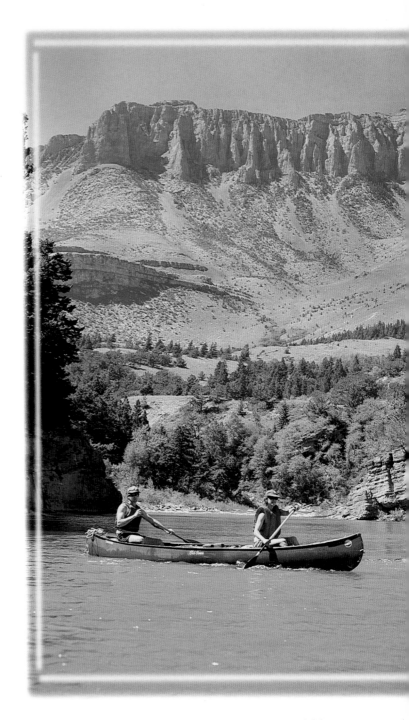

"Every age has its pleasures, its style of wit, and its own ways."

Nicolas Boileau-
Despreaux

What began with a catalog of physical and mental health benefits associated with the active life now concludes with a consideration of the contribution of physical activity to that elusive concept, the quality of life. I'll begin with a consideration of quality and ways to measure it as well as success in life. Then we'll consider how the definition of success shifts with the seasons of life. I'll conclude with an invitation to action, a challenge to maintain and improve the quality of life in your community.

■ This chapter will help you

- construct your definition of quality and success in life,
- understand how the definitions change at different stages of life,
- find ways to influence the quality of your experiences,
- understand your responsibility to maintain and improve the quality of life, and
- appreciate the dimensions of the active life.

Quality of Life

Quality of life, quality time—just what is this quality thing all about? The dictionary definition of quality includes: "degree of excellence"; "a distinguishing attribute." Quality is necessarily a subjective, personal response, not an absolute. Quality is easily distinguished from quantity. For example, for competitive runners, quantity of training simply refers to the miles run, whereas quality refers to the race-pace training that leads to improvement in performance. Similarly, while some find quality in a difficult mountain climb, others prefer the tranquility of a hike in the forest below.

Quality Time

A recent addition to the lexicon of pop-psych, *quality time*, or QT, usually refers to time spent with loved ones. Its value is that it reminds us to do the obvious: spend time with those we value. But QT means more than just spending time; it means being there in mind as well as body. Put aside work or diversions; turn off the cell phone, pager, and TV; and become fully engaged in the moment. Play games with the kids, walk and talk with your significant other, or simply sit and watch the sunset. Don't wait for an accident, heart attack, or some other disaster to remind you of the things that really matter in life.

Objective measurement of this subjective concept has just begun. Research has provided some insights into the relationship between physical activity and the quality of life. Active individuals have better health, more stamina, more positive attitudes toward work, and a greater ability to cope with stress. Active older adults report greater life satisfaction, less dependence on others, and better overall health (Weinberg and Gould 1999). The health care debate has prompted discussion of quality-of-life issues in reference to treatment decisions, such as surgery, chemotherapy, radiation, or drugs. Will surgery or some other therapy improve the quality of life? Removal of the prostate gland may excise a cancer, but it often comes at a terrible cost (incontinence, impotence).

You make quality-of-life decisions daily. Make certain you understand the options and the factors that contribute to your personal definition of quality. Do you value family or friends above wealth and fame, excitement over tranquility, sociability above privacy? Try to be certain that your decisions are consistent with the things you value. To do this you'll have to arrive at your own definition of what constitutes a successful life.

Success

Definitions of success differ among individuals and may change as one ages. Many people set out to be successful in business or a profession, or to earn wealth and fame. In time the definition may be modified to include financial security and more time with family and friends. Consider the things you associate with success.

Remember the lyric "Fame—if you win it, comes and goes in a minute." You don't need fame, status, power, or a pile of money to be successful, just a favorable or satisfactory outcome or result. Few of us look back and wish we had spent more time working or acquiring wealth, whereas many of us wish we had spent more time with family and friends, or in healthy pursuits. Your definition of success may have a lot to do with how you view the quality of life.

The inane bumper sticker "He who has the most toys wins" describes the credo of the motorized recreationist, owner of powerboat, jet ski, all-terrain vehicle, motorcycle, and snowmobile. Though these methods of transportation have a legitimate purpose—access to recreation or work—they have become an end instead of a means. One loud, polluting machine can spoil the tranquility of lake or forest, ruining the quality of experience for human-powered paddlers, hikers, mountain bikers, and cross-country skiers. Worse yet is the realization that this lifestyle is being handed down to the next generation of overweight, underactive kids.

> Remember the lyric "Fame—if you win it, comes and goes in a minute."

Healthy, Wealthy, and Wise

For years we have known that physical activity is associated with education and income. Does that mean that becoming active will increase your intelligence, or your income? Probably not, but a recent study that compared the connection between health and success among leaders of some of America's top 100 corporations to the average American citizen found that the corporate execs weighed 12 pounds (5.4 kilograms) less; ate more fish and salad; consumed less coffee, alcohol, or tobacco; and stayed married longer. And they named exercise as their number-one form of stress management (Edstrom 1999).

Perception of Quality

Psychologists and sensory physiologists long have known how to measure the quantity of stimulus (e.g., sound, light, exertion). It is far more difficult to assess the quality of an experience, yet it is the quality of an exercise experience that provides pleasure and brings us back for more. Ask someone to rate the quality of an exercise experience, and he or she will respond with a long-winded evaluation of the physical environment, weather, companions, personal sensations, expectations. Many factors are involved in the quality of an exercise experience.

A creek-side run on a tree-shaded path amid the beauty of the mountains is an experience to be savored and long remembered. Cover the same distance on a short, crowded running track or along a busy city street, and the experience becomes an ordeal, unless, of course, you are with company you enjoy, or glad for the chance to get away from the office. You can control the factors that enhance the quality of your exercise experiences. If you abhor noisy, crowded public tennis courts and are bothered by players who either don't know or won't practice the etiquette of the sport, build your own court, join a private club, play before the crowds arrive, or encourage the city recreation department to teach court etiquette. Your exercise experiences will be more enjoyable if you follow these guidelines:

- **Be flexible:** Don't depend on one activity, time, or place for satisfaction.
- **Plan ahead:** Plan your participation, your companions, the time of day, the place. If the afternoon winds diminish the quality of tennis, plan to play in the morning.
- **Set realistic goals:** If you set out to run 10 miles (16 kilometers) on a hot, humid day and don't finish, you may feel that you've failed, but you haven't. You just set an unrealistic goal.
- **Recognize your moods:** We all get depressed, concerned, worried. Sometimes exercise can help you calm down when you're too excited or pick you up when you're depressed, but a really foul mood can ruin the experience for you and your companion.
- **Be prepared:** Keep your equipment in good condition, get adequate rest, eat sensibly, bring extra food or drink if it may be needed, and have first aid supplies, tools, and extra parts available.
- **Learn to relax:** Sit in a quiet room and focus on your respiration. Think "easy" with each exhale. Practice daily, and when you become proficient, start using the technique in your sport, while driving in traffic, or whenever the need arises.

It is up to you to ensure the quality of your exercise experiences. If your daily activity is satisfying, it may bubble over and affect other phases of life. If it isn't, you may feel cheated, lose interest in the activity, and quit. In that case, you will be the loser.

The Seasons and Stages of Life

Physical activity should be spontaneous and enjoyable. Excessive planning can inhibit spontaneity and induce the kind of drudgery found in many fitness programs. On the other hand, a well-conceived plan can contribute to the flow of life, helping one season melt into the other. Just this once, give your physical life the same attention you give to work, finances, education, or travel. We'll look first at the seasons of the year, then the stages of life.

Annual Plan

Once a year take the time to outline the activities in which you intend to participate during the coming year. Fill in the sports or recreational activities you enjoy each season. When you come upon a blank season, consider a new activity, a supplement, or preparation for an upcoming season (figure 20.1). This brief exercise will also show you how one activity can blend into the next, removing the need for extensive physical preparation. Arm endurance developed in swimming transfers to cross-country ski poling and then to paddling a canoe. Year-round activity is the ideal way to maintain a desired level of fitness; it minimizes the discomfort associated with the first few days of exercise, maintains fitness, and optimizes energy balance. Of course, most of us remain active because we enjoy the experiences.

Give some thought to activities you want to take up in the future, when you'll have the time to enjoy them.

Stages of Life

Each of us is engaged in a lifelong search for meaning. The seasons of our lives are marked by an ebb and flow of purpose and confidence, periods of satisfaction followed by doubt. Our goals shift as the stages unfold.

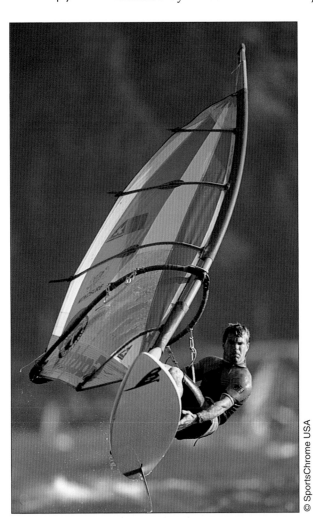

The stages of life provide many challenges and opportunities.

- **Young adult:** This stage usually requires severing ties, acquiring an education, finding a mate, establishing a career, and perhaps starting a family. So it isn't surprising to find definitions of success framed in financial and material terms.

- **Adult:** By avoiding divorce and major career changes, the 30-something adult may be able to purchase a home and put down roots. But that goal is often threatened by uncertainties in the workplace or the economy. And this period sometimes brings the midlife crisis, a realization that time to reach goals is running out.

During the decade from 45 to 55 years, what some call *middle age,* we begin to accept ourselves and our lives, and to redefine our goals for success and the quality of life. Thereafter we may be refreshed or resigned, facing the best time of life if we let go of old roles and definitions and find a renewal of purpose (Sheehy 1976).

- **Senior:** Sometimes called the golden years, the senior stage may be the best of all, finally providing the time and resources to fulfill personal goals. Limited resources won't diminish satisfaction if the goals are qualitative rather than quantitative.

Seasonal Activity Planner

	Winter	Spring	Summer	Fall
Major activities				
Minor activities				
Supplements				

Figure 20.1 Seasonal activity planner.

• **Elder:** Sometime after the age of 80 folks say they begin to slow down but not stop. Many artists and musicians continue to create and perform. In spite of crippling rheumatoid arthritis, my independent mother continued to play the piano in musical programs until shortly before her death at the age of 84. Gardening and swimming helped maintain the physical vitality she needed to pursue her passion for music.

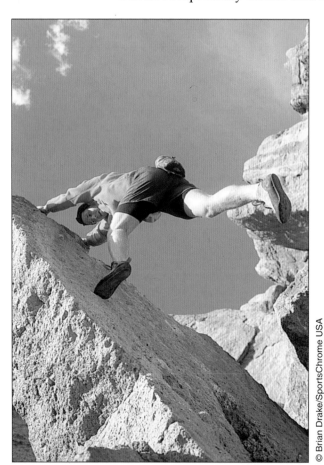

Remain open to peak experiences and flow.

© Brian Drake/SportsChrome USA

Too busy to do all the things you want to do? Some activities, such as football, should be attempted only by the young, whereas others are perfectly suited for adults, seniors, or even elders. Activities such as fishing, sailing, or golf can be enjoyed at any stage of life. So relax; there is time for everything you want to do. Give some thought to activities you want to take up in the future, when you'll have the time to enjoy them.

As you advance in years you will find new challenges and new adventures, and although you may temporarily put aside favorite activities, you'll never forget well-learned skills. Competition becomes more difficult as you approach the top of an age group, but when you enter a new age classification, it's like being a kid again. Eventually, most of us seek less competition and more cooperation; we discover the quiet

Glossary

acclimatization—Adaptation to an environmental condition such as heat or altitude

actin—Muscle protein that works with the protein myosin to produce movement

adenosine triphosphate (ATP)—High-energy compound formed from oxidation of fat and carbohydrate, used as energy supply for muscle and other body functions; the energy currency

adipose tissue—Tissue in which fat is stored

aerobic—In the presence of oxygen; aerobic metabolism utilizes oxygen

aerobic fitness—Maximum ability to take in, transport, and utilize oxygen

agility—Ability to change direction quickly while maintaining control of the body

alveoli—Tiny air sacs in the lungs where oxygen and carbon dioxide exchange takes place

amino acids—Chief components of proteins; different arrangements of the 22 amino acids form the various proteins (muscles, enzymes, hormones, etc.)

anaerobic—In the absence of oxygen; nonoxidation metabolism

anaerobic threshold—More properly called the lactate threshold, the point at which lactic acid produced in muscles begins to accumulate in the blood; defines the upper limit that can be sustained aerobically

angina pectoris—Chest pain (also called necktie pain) associated with narrowed coronary arteries and lack of oxygen to heart muscle during exertion

anorexia nervosa—An eating disorder characterized by excessive dieting and subsequent loss of appetite

arrhythmia—Irregular rhythm or beat of the heart

asymptomatic—Without symptoms

atherosclerosis—Narrowing of coronary arteries by cholesterol buildup within the walls

atrophy—Loss of size of muscle

balance—Ability to maintain equilibrium while in motion

behavior therapy—A system of record keeping and motivation designed to help change a behavior (e.g., overeating)

blood pressure—Force exerted against the walls of arteries

body composition—The relative amounts of fat and lean tissue

bronchiole—Small branch of airway; sometimes undergoes spasm, making breathing difficult, as in exercise-induced asthma

buffer—Substance in blood that soaks up hydrogen ions to minimize changes in acid-base balance (pH)

bulimia—An eating disorder characterized by alternate bouts of gorging and purging

calorie—Amount of heat required to raise one kilogram of water one degree Celsius; same as kilocalorie

capillaries—Smallest blood vessels (between arterioles and venules) where oxygen, foods, and hormones are delivered to tissues and carbon dioxide and wastes are picked up

carbohydrate—Simple (e.g., sugar) and complex (e.g., potatoes, rice, beans, corn, and grains) foodstuff that we use for energy; stored in liver and muscle as glycogen, while excess can be stored as fat

cardiac—Pertaining to the heart

cardiac output—Volume of blood pumped by the heart each minute; product of heart rate and stroke volume

cardiorespiratory endurance—Synonymous with aerobic fitness or maximal oxygen intake

cardiovascular system—Heart and blood vessels

central nervous system (CNS)—The brain and spinal cord

cholesterol—Fatty substance found in nerves and other tissues; excessive amounts in blood have been associated with increased risk of heart disease

Clo units—The insulating value of clothing

concentric—Contraction that involves shortening of the contracted muscle

contraction—Development of tension by muscle: concentric muscle shortens and eccentric muscle lengthens under tension; static contractions are contractions without change in length

cool-down—Postperformance exercise used to dissipate heat, maintain blood flow, and aid recovery of muscles

coronary arteries—Blood vessels that originate from the aorta and branch out to supply oxygen and fuels to the heart muscle

coronary-prone—Having several risk factors related to the development of heart disease

creatine phosphate (CP)—Energy-rich compound that backs up ATP in providing energy for muscles

defibrillator—Device that applies a strong electric shock to stop irregular heart action and restore normal heart rhythm

dehydration—Loss of essential body fluids

delayed onset muscle soreness (DOMS)—Muscle soreness that peaks 24 to 48 hours after unfamiliar exercise or vigorous eccentric contractions

deoxyribonucleic acid (DNA)—The source of the genetic code housed in the nucleus of the cell

detraining—Cessation of training; used to observe the decline of important measures (e.g., blood volume) associated with performance

diastolic pressure—Lowest pressure exerted by blood in an artery; occurs during the resting phase (diastole) of the heart cycle

dieting—Eating according to a prescribed plan

duration—Distance or length of time (or calories burned, in the case of the exercise prescription)

eccentric—Contraction that involves lengthening of a contracted muscle

electrocardiogram (ECG)—A graphic recording of the electrical activity of the heart

electrolyte—Solution of ions (sodium, potassium) that conducts electric current

endurance—The ability to persist or to resist fatigue

energy balance—Balance of caloric intake and expenditure

enzyme—An organic catalyst that accelerates the rate of chemical reactions

epinephrine (adrenaline)—Hormone from the adrenal medulla and nerve endings of the sympathetic nervous system; secreted during times of stress and to help mobilize energy

ergometer—A device, such as a bicycle, used to measure work capacity

evaporation—Elimination of body heat when sweat vaporizes on the surface of the skin; evaporation of one liter of sweat yields a heat loss of 580 calories

Fartlek—Swedish term meaning speed play; a form of training in which participants vary speed according to mood as they run through the countryside

fast-twitch muscle fibers—Muscle fibers that contract quickly but are susceptible to fatigue

fat—Important energy source; stored for future use when excess calories are ingested

fatigue—Diminished work capacity, usually short of true physiological limits; real limits in short, intense exercise are factors within muscle (muscle pH, calcium); in long-duration effort, limits are glycogen depletion or central nervous system fatigue due in part to low blood sugar

fitness—A combination of aerobic capacity and muscular strength and endurance that enhances health, performance, and the quality of life

flexibility—Range of motion through which the limbs or body parts are able to move

frequency—Number of times per day or week (in the case of the exercise prescription)

glucose—Energy source transported in blood; essential energy source for brain and nervous tissue

glycemic index—A measure of how rapidly a carbohydrate is digested and absorbed into the blood

glycogen—Storage form of glucose; found in liver and muscles

heart attack—Death of heart muscle tissue that results when atherosclerosis blocks oxygen delivery to heart muscle; also called myocardial infarction

heart rate—Frequency of contraction, often inferred from pulse rate (expansion of artery resulting from beat of heart)

heart rate range—The difference between the resting and maximal heart rates

heat stress—Temperature-humidity combination that leads to heat disorders such as heat cramps, heat exhaustion, or heatstroke

hemoglobin—Iron-containing compound in red blood cells that forms a loose association with oxygen

high-density lipoprotein (HDL) cholesterol—A carrier molecule that takes cholesterol from the tissue to the liver for removal; inversely related to heart disease risk

hyperthermia—An alarming rise in body temperature that sets the stage for heat stress disorders

hypoglycemia—Low blood sugar (glucose)

hypothermia—Life-threatening heat loss brought on by rapid cooling, energy depletion, and exhaustion

inhibition—Opposite of excitation in the nervous system

insulin—Pancreatic hormone responsible for getting blood sugar into cells

intensity—The relative rate, speed, or level of exertion

interval training—Training method that alternates short bouts of intense effort with periods of active rest

ischemia—Lack of blood to a specific area such as heart muscle

isokinetic—Contraction against resistance that is varied to maintain high tension throughout range of motion

isometric—Contraction against an immovable object (static contraction)

isotonic—Contraction against a constant resistance

lactic acid—A by-product of glycogen metabolism that also transports energy from muscle to muscle and from muscle to the liver; high levels in muscle poison the contractile apparatus and inhibit enzyme activity

lean body weight—Body weight minus fat weight

lipid—Fat

lipoprotein—A fat-protein complex that serves as a carrier in the blood (e.g., high-density lipoprotein cholesterol)

low-density lipoprotein (LDL) cholesterol—The cholesterol fraction that accumulates in the lining of the coronary arteries and causes ischemia

maximal oxygen intake (consumption)—Aerobic fitness; measure of fitness with implications for health; synonymous with $\dot{V}O_2$max and cardiorespiratory fitness

metabolic equivalent (MET)—Unit of measure; one MET is resting metabolism

metabolism—Energy production and utilization processes, often mediated by enzymatic pathways

mitochondria—Tiny organelles within cells; site of all oxidative energy production

motoneuron—Nerve that transmits impulses to muscle fibers

motor area—Portion of cerebral cortex that controls movement

motor unit—Motor nerve and the muscle fibers it innervates

muscle fiber types—Fast-twitch fibers are fast contracting but fast to fatigue; slow-twitch fibers contract somewhat more slowly but are fatigue-resistant

muscular endurance—The ability to sustain muscular contractions

muscular fitness—The strength, muscular endurance, and flexibility needed to carry out daily tasks and avoid injury

myocardium—Heart muscle

myofibril—Contractile threads of muscle composed of the proteins actin and myosin

myogenic—Training that influences the muscles

myosin—Muscle protein that works with actin to produce movement

neurogenic—Training that influences the nervous system

neuron—Nerve cell that conducts an impulse; basic unit of the nervous system

nutrition—Provision of adequate energy (calories) as well as needed amounts of fat, carbohydrate, protein, vitamins, minerals, and water

obesity—Excessive body fat (more than 20 percent of total body weight for men, more than 30 percent for women)

osteoporosis—Weakening of bones via the loss of bone minerals

overload—A greater load than normally experienced; used to coax a training effect from the body

overtraining—Excess training that leads to staleness, illness, or injury

oxygen debt—Postexercise oxygen intake that exceeds resting requirements; used to replace the oxygen deficit incurred during exercise

oxygen deficit—Lack of oxygen in early moments of exercise

oxygen intake—Oxygen used to provide energy via oxidative pathways

perceived exertion—Subjective estimate of exercise difficulty

peripheral nervous system—Parts of the nervous system not including the brain and spinal cord

pH—Acidity or alkalinity of a solution; below 7 is acid, and above 7 is alkaline

physiological age—Also called functional age; as contrasted to chronological age, defines an individual's ability to perform physically

Keul, J. 1971. Myocardial metabolism in athletes. In *Muscle metabolism during exercise,* ed. B. Pemow and B. Saltin. New York: Plenum.

Kline, G., J. Pocari, R. Hintermeister, P. Freedson, A. Ward, R. McCarron, J. Ross, and J. Rippe. 1987. Estimation of $\dot{V}O_2$max from a one-mile track walk, gender, age, and body weight. *Medicine and Science in Sports and Exercise* 19:253-59.

Klissouras, V. 1976. Heritability of adaptive variation. *Journal of Applied Physiology* 31:338-44.

Kobasa, S. 1979. Stressful life events, personality and health: An inquiry into hardiness. *Journal of Personality and Social Psychology* 37:1-11.

Komi, P. 1992. Stretch-shortening cycle. In *Strength and power in sport,* ed. P. Komi. Oxford: Blackwell Scientific.

Komi, P., and E.R. Buskirk. 1972. Effect of eccentric and concentric muscle conditioning on tension and electrical activity of human muscle. *Ergonomics* 15:417-22.

Kramer, J., M. Stone, H. Obryant, M. Conley, R. Johnson, D. Nieman, D. Honeycutt, and T. Hoke. 1997. Effects of single vs multiple sets of weight training: Impact of volume, intensity and variation. *Journal of Strength and Conditioning Research* 11:143-47.

Kramsch, D., A. Aspen, B. Abramowitz, T. Kreimendahl, and W. Hood. 1981. Reduction of coronary atherosclerosis by moderate conditioning exercise in monkeys on an atherogenic diet. *New England Journal of Medicine* 305:1483-89.

Kraus, H., and W. Raab. 1961. *Hypokinetic disease.* Springfield, IL: Charles C Thomas.

Lakka, T., J. Venalainen, R. Rauramaa, R. Salonen, J. Tuomilehto, and J. Salonen. 1994. Relation of leisure-time physical activity and cardiorespiratory fitness to the risk of acute myocardial infarction in men. *New England Journal of Medicine* 330:1549-54.

Landers, D., and S. Petruzzello. 1994. Physical activity, fitness and anxiety. In *Physical activity, fitness and health,* ed. C. Bouchard, R. Shephard, and T. Stevens. Champaign, IL: Human Kinetics.

Landy, F. 1992. Alternatives to chronological age in determining standards of suitability for public safety jobs, vol. 1. Tech. Rep. Pennsylvania State University.

Leaf, A. 1973. Getting old. *Scientific American* 229:45-55.

Lee, C., A. Jackson, and S. Blair. 1998. U.S. Weight Guidelines: Is it also important to consider cardiorespiratory fitness? *International Journal of Obesity* 22(Suppl.):2-7.

Lee, I-Min, C. Hsieh, and R. Paffenbarger. 1995. Exercise intensity and longevity in men: The Harvard alumni health study. *Journal of the American Medical Association* 273:1179-84.

Leibel, R., M. Rosenbaum, and J. Hirsch. 1995. Changes in energy expenditure resulting from altered body weight. *New England Journal of Medicine* 332:621-28.

Leitzmann, M., E. Rimm, W. Willett, D. Spiegelman, F. Grodstein, M. Stampfer, G. Colditz, and E. Giovannucci. 1999. Recreational physical activity and the risk of cholecystectomy in women. *New England Journal of Medicine* 341:777-84.

Lemon, P. 1995. Do athletes need more protein and amino acids? *International Journal of Sports and Nutrition* 5:S39-S61.

Leon, A., J. Connett, D. Jacobs, and R. Rauramaa. 1987. Leisure-time physical activity levels and risk of coronary heart disease and death: The multiple risk factor intervention trial. *Journal of the American Medical Association* 258:2388-95.

Leonard, J., J. Hofer, and N. Pritikin. 1974. *Live longer now.* Mountain View, CA: World Sports Library.

Libonati, J. 1999. Myocardial diastolic function and exercise. *Medicine and Science in Sports and Exercise* 31:1741-47.

Lieber, C. 1976. The metabolism of alcohol. *Scientific American* 229: 45-55.

Locke, E., and G. Latham. 1985. The application of goal setting to sports. *Journal of Sports Psychology* 7:205-22.

Lopez, S.A., R. Vial, L. Balart, and G. Arroyave. 1974. Effects of exercise and physical fitness on serum lipids and lipoproteins. *Atherosclerosis* 20:1-9.

Lubell, A. 1988. Blacks and exercise. *The Physician and Sportsmedicine* 16:162-76.

Mackinnon, L. 1992. *Exercise and immunology.* Champaign, IL: Human Kinetics.

Madden, L.B. 2000. Muscle as a consumer of lactate. *Medicine and Science in Sports and Exercise* 32:764-71.

Malina, R., and C. Bouchard. 1991. *Growth, maturation, and physical activity.* Champaign, IL: Human Kinetics.

Malmivaara, A., U. Hakkinen, T. Aro, M. Heinrichs, L. Koskenniemi, E. Kuosma, S. Lappi, R. Paloheimo, C. Servo, V. Vaaranen, and S. Hernberg. 1995. The treatment of acute low back pain: Bed rest, exercises, or ordinary activity? *New England Journal of Medicine* 332:351-55.

Manson, J., F. Hu, J. Rich-Edwards, G. Colditz, M. Stampfer, W. Willet, F. Speizer, and C. Hennekens. 1999. A prospective study of walking as compared with vigorous exercise in the prevention of coronary heart disease in women, *New England Journal of Medicine* 341:650-58.

Manson, J., W. Willett, M. Stampfer, G. Colditz, D. Hunter, S. Hankinson, C. Hennekens, and F. Speizer. 1995. Body weight and mortality among women. *New England Journal of Medicine* 333:677-85.

Markoff, R., P. Ryan, and T. Young. 1982. Endorphins and mood changes in long-distance running. *Medicine and Science in Sports and Exercise* 14(1):11-15.

Maslow, A.H. 1954. *Motivation and personality.* New York: Harper.

Massey, B.H., R.C. Nelson, B.J. Sharkey, and T. Comden. 1965. Effects of high-frequency electrical stimulation on the size and strength of skeletal muscle. *Journal of Sports Medicine* 5:136-44.

Matejek, N., E. Weimann, C. Witzel, G. Molenkamp, S. Schwidergall, and H. Bohles. 1999. Hypoleptinaemia in patients with anorexia nervosa and in elite gymnasts with anorexia athletica. *International Journal of Sports Medicine* 20:451-56.

Mayer, J., and B.A. Bullen. 1974. Nutrition, weight control and exercise. In *Science and medicine of exercise and sport,* ed. W.R. Johnson and E.R. Buskirk. New York: Harper and Row.

McArdle, W., F. Katch, and V. Katch. 1994. *Essentials of exercise physiology.* Philadelphia: Lea & Febiger.

McAuley, E., and B. Blissmer. 2000. Self-efficacy determinants and consequences of physical activity. In *Exercise and sports science reviews,* Vol. 28, ed. D. Seals, 85-88. Indianapolis: American College of Sports Medicine.

Miller, D., and P. Payne. 1968. Longevity and protein intake. *Experimental Gerontology* 3:231-35.

Mitchell, J.H., W. Reardon, D.I. McCloskey, and K. Wildnethal. 1977. Possible roles of muscle receptors in the cardiovascular response to exercise. In *The marathon,* ed. P. Milvy, 232-52. New York: New York Academy of Sciences.

Móle, P.A., K.M. Baldwin, R.L. Terjung, and J.O. Holloszy. 1973. Enzymatic pathways of pyruvate metabolism in skeletal muscle: Adaptations to exercise. *American Journal of Physiology* 224:50-54.

Móle, P.A., L.B. Oscai, and J.O. Holloszy. 1971. Adaptation of muscle to exercise: Increase in levels of palmityl CoA synthetase, carnitine palmityl-transferase, and palmityl CoA dehydrogenase, and in the capacity to oxidize fatty acids. *Journal of Clinical Investigation* 50:2323-29.

Móle, P.A., J. Stern, C. Schultz, E. Bernauer, and B. Holcomb. 1989. Exercise reverses depressed metabolic rate produced by severe caloric restriction. *Medicine and Science in Sports and Exercise* 21:29-33.

Molz, A., B. Heyduck, H. Lill, E. Spanuth, and L. Rocker. 1993. The effect of different exercise intensities on the fibrinolytic system. *European Journal of Applied Physiology and Occupational Physiology* 67:298-304.

Montner, P., Y. Zou, R. Robergs, G. Murata, D. Stark, C. Quinn, and J. Greene. 1995. Mechanism of glycerol-induced fluid retention and heartrate reduction during exercise. *Medicine and Science in Sports and Exercise* 27:S19.

Morgan, W.P. 1979. Negative addiction in runners. *The Physician and Sportsmedicine* 7:57-70.

Morgan, W.P., and S. Goldston. 1987. *Exercise and mental health.* New York: Hemisphere.

Morgan, W., P. O'Conner, A. Ellickson, and P. Bradley. 1988. Personality structure, mood states and performance in elite male distance runners. *International Journal of Sport Psychology* 19:247-63.

Morrey, M., and D. Hensrud. 1999. Risk of medical events in a supervised health and fitness facility. *Medicine and Science in Sports and Exercise* 31:1233-36.

Morris, J., and M. Crawford. 1958. Coronary heart disease and physical activity of work. *Journal of the British Medical Association* 2:1485-96.

Morris, J.N., and P. Raffle. 1954. Coronary heart disease in transport workers. *British Journal of Industrial Medicine* 11:260-72.

Morrissey, M., E. Harman, and M. Johnson. 1995. Resistance training modes: Specificity and effectiveness. *Medicine and Science in Sports and Exercise* 27:648-60.

Nadel, E.R., ed. 1977. *Problems with temperature regulation during exercise.* New York: Academic Press.

Neary, J., G. Wheeler, I. Maclean, D. Cumming, and H. Quinney. 1994. Urinary free cortisol as an indicator of exercise training stress. *Clinical Journal of Sports Medicine* 4:160-65.

Nelson, M., M. Fiatarone, C. Morganti, I. Trice, R. Greenberg, and W. Evans. 1994. Effects of high-intensity strength training on multiple risk factors for osteoporotic fractures: A randomized controlled trial. *Journal of the American Medical Association* 272:1909-14.

Newham, D. 1988. The consequences of eccentric contractions and their relationship to delayed onset muscle pain. *European Journal of Applied Physiology* 57:353-59.

Nieman, D. 1998. Immunity in athletics: Current issues. *Sports Science Exchange* 11(2). Chicago: Gatorade Sports Science Institute.

Nieman, D., and B. Pedersen. 1999. Exercise and immune function: Recent developments. *Sports Medicine* 27:73-80.

Nikkila, E., M. Taskinen, S. Rehunen, and M. Harkonen. 1978. Lipoprotein lipase activity in adipose tissue and skeletal muscle of runners: Relationship to serum lipoproteins. *Metabolism* 27:1661-67.

North, T., P. McCullagh, and Z.V. Tran. 1990. Effects of exercise on depression. *Exercise and Sport Science Reviews* 18:379-415.

Ornish, D. 1993. *Eat more, weigh less.* New York: Harper Collins.

Ornstein, R., and D. Sobel. 1989. *Healthy pleasures.* New York: Addison-Wesley.

Oscai, L.B., and J.O. Holloszy. 1969. Effects of weight changes produced by exercise, food restriction or overeating on body composition. *Journal of Clinical Investigation* 48:2124-28.

Paffenbarger, R. 1978. Physical activity as an index of heart disease risk in college alumni. *American Journal of Epidemiology* 108:161-72.

Paffenbarger, R. 1994. Forty years of progress: Physical activity, health and fitness. In *American College of Sports Medicine 40th anniversary lectures,* 93-109. Indianapolis.

Paffenbarger, R., R. Hyde, and A. Wing. 1986. Physical activity, all-cause mortality, and longevity of college alumni. *New England Journal of Medicine* 314:605-13.

Paffenbarger, R., R. Hyde, and A. Wing. 1990. Physical activity and physical fitness as determinants of health and longevity. In *Exercise, fitness, and health,* ed. C. Bouchard, R.J. Shephard, T. Stephens, J.R. Sutton, and B.D. McPherson. Champaign, IL: Human Kinetics.

Passmore, R., and J. Durnin. 1955. Human energy expenditure. *Physiology Review* 35:801-24.

Pate, R., M. Pratt, S. Blair, W. Haskell, C. Macera, C. Bouchard, D. Buchner, W. Ettinger, G. Heath, A. King, A. Kriska, A. Leon, B. Marcus, J. Morris, R. Paffenbarger, K. Patrick, M. Pollock, J. Rippe, J. Sallis, and J. Wilmore. 1995. Physical activity and public health: A recommendation from the Centers for Disease Control and Prevention and the American College of Sports Medicine. *Journal of the American Medical Association* 273:402-7.

Pedersen, B., J. Helge, E. Richter, T. Rohde, and B. Kiens. 2000. Training and natural immunity: Effects of diets rich in fat or carbohydrate. *European Journal of Applied Physiology* 82:98-103.

Pette, D. 1984. Activity induced fast to slow transitions in mammalian muscle. *Medicine and Science in Sports and Exercise* 16:517-28.

Piers, L., M. Soares, L. McCormack, and K. O'Dea. 1998. Is there evidence for an age-related reduction in metabolic rate? *Journal of Applied Physiology* 85:2196-2204.

Plunkett, B., and W. Hopkins. 1995. The cause and treatment of the side pain "stitch". *Medicine and Science in Sports and Exercise* 27:S23.

Pollock, M.L. 1973. The quantification of endurance training programs. In *Exercise and sports sciences reviews,* vol. 1, ed. J.H. Wilmore. New York: Academic Press.

Pollock, M.L., J. Dimmick, H. Miller, Z. Kendrick, and A. Linnerud. 1975. Effects of mode of training on cardiovascular function and body composition of middle-aged men. *Medicine and Science in Sports and Exercise* 7:139-45.

Pomerleau, O., H. Scherzer, N. Grunberg, C. Pomerleau, J. Judge, J. Fertig, and J. Burleson. 1987. The effects of acute exercise on subsequent cigarette smoking. *Journal of Behavioral Medicine* 10(2):117-27.

Powel, K., and R. Paffenbarger. 1985. Workshop on epidemiologic and public health aspects of physical activity and exercise: A summary. *Public Health Reports* 100:118-26.

President's Council on Physical Fitness and Sport. 1973, May. National adult physical fitness survey. *PCPFandS Newsletter*, 1-27.

President's Council on Physical Fitness and Sport. 1975. *An introduction to physical fitness.* Washington, D.C.: President's Council on Physical Fitness and Sport.

Pritikin, N. 1979. *The Pritikin program for diet and exercise.* New York: Bantam.

Puchkoff, J., L. Curry, J. Swan, B. Sharkey, and B. Ruby. 1998. The effects of hydration status and blood glucose on mental performance during extended exercise in the heat. *Medicine and Science in Sports and Exercise* 30:S284.

Raab, W. 1965. Prevention of ischaemic heart disease. *Medical Services Journal of Canada* 21:719-34.

Radcliffe, J., and R. Farentinos. 1985. *Plyometrics: Explosive power training.* Champaign, IL: Human Kinetics.

Rejeski, W., K. Neal, M. Wurst, P. Brubaker, and W. Ettinger Jr. 1995. Walking, but not weight lifting, acutely reduces systolic blood pressure in older sedentary men and women. *Journal of Aging and Physical Activity* 3:163-77.

Ridker, P., C. Hennekens, J. Buring, and N. Rifai. 2000. C-reactive protein and other markers of inflammation in the prediction of cardiovascular disease in women. *New England Journal of Medicine* 342:836-43.

Rising, R., I. Harper, A. Fontvielle, R. Ferraro, M. Spraul, and E. Ravussin. 1994. Determinants of total daily energy expenditure: Variability in physical activity. *American Journal of Clinical Nutrition* 59:800-804.

Ross, R., H. Pedwell, and J. Rissanen. 1995. Effects of energy restriction and exercise on skeletal muscle and adipose tissue in women as measured by magnetic resonance imaging. *American Journal of Clinical Nutrition* 61:1179-85.

Roth, D., and D. Holmes. 1985. Influence of physical fitness in determining the impact of stressful life events on physical and psychological health. *Psychosomatic Medicine* 47:164-73.

Roth, E.M., ed. 1968. *Compendium of human responses to the aerospace environment III.* Washington, D.C.: National Aeronautics and Space Administration.

Ruby, B., and R. Robergs. 1994. Gender differences in substrate utilization during exercise. *Sports Medicine* 17:393-410.

Ruby, B., D. Schoeller, and B. Sharkey. 2001. Evaluation of total energy expenditure (doubly-labeled water) across different measurement periods during arduous work. *Medicine and Science in Sports and Exercise* 33:S274.

Ryan, A., R. Pratley, D. Elahi, and A. Goldberg. 1995. Resistive training increases fat-free mass and maintains RMR despite weight loss in postmenopausal women. *Journal of Applied Physiology* 79:818-23.

Ryder, H.W., H.J. Carr, and R. Herget. 1976. Future performance in footracing. *Scientific American* 234:109-16.

Saltin, B. 1977. The interplay between peripheral and central factors in the adaptive response to exercise and training. In *The marathon,* ed. P. Milvy, 224-31. New York: New York Academy of Sciences.

Saltin, B., G. Blomqvist, J.H. Mitchell, R.L. Johnson Jr., K. Wildenthal, and C.B. Chapman. 1968. Response to exercise after bed rest and after training. *Circulation* 38(Suppl. 7):1-78.

Seltzer, C.C., and J. Mayer. 1965. A simple criterion of obesity. *Postgraduate Medicine* 38:A101-106.

Selye, H. 1956. *The stress of life.* New York: McGraw-Hill.

Sharkey, B.J. 1970. Intensity and duration of training and the development of cardiorespiratory endurance. *Medicine and Science in Sports and Exercise* 2:197-202.

Sharkey, B.J. 1974. *Physiological fitness and weight control.* Missoula, MT: Mountain Press.

Sharkey, B.J. 1975. *Physiology and physical activity.* New York: Harper and Row.

Index

Note: Tables and figures are indicated with an italicized *t* or *f*.

About the Author

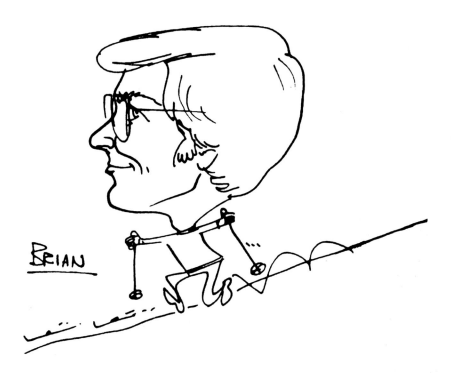

BRIAN

Brian J. Sharkey brings more than 35 years experience as a leading fitness researcher, educator, and consultant to his latest work. He was president of the American College of Sports Medicine in 1991 and 1992. He has also researched the relationship of exercise physiology to consumers' daily health habits.

Director of the University of Montana's Human Performance Laboratory for many years, Sharkey remains associated with the university and lab as professor emeritus. Sharkey also works with the U.S. Forest Service as a consultant in the areas of fitness, health, and work capacity. He received the U.S. Department of Agriculture's Superior Service Award in 1977 and its Distinguished Service Award in 1993 for his contributions to the health, safety, and performance of firefighters.

In his leisure time, Sharkey enjoys cross-country skiing, mountain biking, running, hiking, and canoeing. He and his wife, Barbara, live in Missoula, Montana.

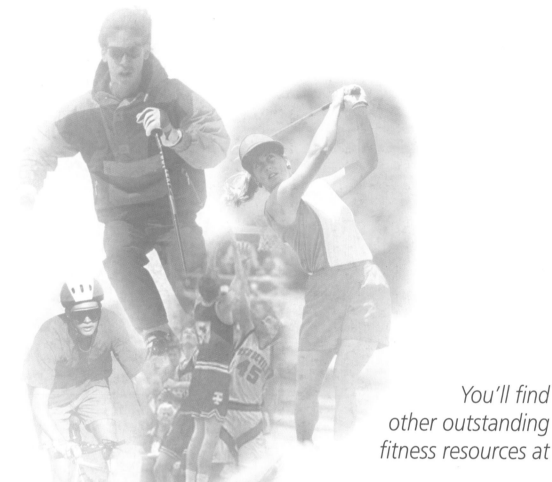

*You'll find
other outstanding
fitness resources at*

www.humankinetics.com

In the U.S. cal

1-800-747-4457

Australia	08 8277 1555
Canada	1-800-465-7301
Europe	+44 (0) 113 278 1708
New Zealand	09-523-3462

HUMAN KINETICS
The Information Leader in Physical Activity
P.O. Box 5076 • Champaign, IL 61825-5076 USA